Complementary Medicine
in Australia and New Zealand

Its popularisation, legitimation

and dilemmas

Complementary Medicine in Australia and New Zealand

Its popularisation, legitimation and dilemmas

HANS A. BAER
Development Studies, School of Philosophy,
Anthropology, and Social Inquiry and Centre for Health and
Society University of Melbourne

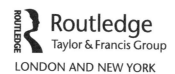
Routledge
Taylor & Francis Group

LONDON AND NEW YORK

First published 2009 by Goshawk Publishing

Published in 2016
by Routledge
2 Park Square, Milton Park, Abingdon, Oxon OX14 4RN
711 Third Avenue, New York, NY, 10017, USA

Routledge is an imprint of the Taylor & Francis Group, an informa business

National Library of Australia Cataloguing-in-Publication data

Baer, Hans A., 1944-
Complementary medicine in Australia and New Zealand : its popularisation,
legitimation and dilemmas / Hans A Baer.

ISBN 13: 9780975742273 (pbk)

Contents

GLOSSARY

ASSOCIATIONS, ORGANISATIONS AND SCHOOLS

AESO	Acupuncture Ethics and Standards Organisation
AACMA	Australian Acupuncture and Chinese Medicine Association
AHA	Australian Herbalists' Association
ACA	Australian Chiropractors' Association
ACHN	Australian College of Holistic Nurses
ACNM	Australian College of Natural Medicine
ACHA	Australian Complementary Health Association
ACMA	Australian Complementary Medical Association
ACNEM	Australian College of Nutritional and Environment Medicine
AMAS	Australian Medical Acupuncture Society
AOA	Australian Osteopathic Association
AMA	Australian Medical Association
ANTA	Australian Natural Therapists Association
ATMS	Australian Traditional-Medicine Society
BMA	British Medical Association
COCA	Chiropractic and Osteopathic College of Australasia
MACCAH	Ministerial Advisory Committee on Complementary and Alternative Health (New Zealand)
NCCAM	National Center for Complementary and Alternative Medicine
NHMRC	National Health and Medical Research Council
NHAA	National Herbalist Association of Australia
NZCA	New Zealand Chiropractic Association
NZMA	New Zealand Medical Association
NZNMA	New Zealand Natural Medicine Association
OCNZ	Osteopathic Council of New Zealand
RCNA	Royal College of Nursing, Australia
SSNT	Southern School of Natural Therapies
TGA	Therapeutic Goods Administration
UCAA	United Chiropractors Association of Australia

PREFACE

*T*he casual visitor to Australia and New Zealand will quickly discover that alternative medicine, complementary medicine, or natural medicine, whatever one may wish to call it, has taken these two countries by storm, just as has been in the case in many other developed societies, particularly ones in North America and Europe. On a walk around Australian and New Zealand cities and even country towns, particularly those closely situated to the capital cities, one will notice offices advertising the services of chiropractors, osteopaths, naturopaths, acupuncturists, Chinese medicine practitioners, massage therapists, Western herbalists, homoeopaths, reflexologists, and sundry other types of heterodox practitioners. One will even notice signs indicating that some conventional or biomedical practitioners offer alternative therapies. The casual visitor on his or her stroll may also notice centres of complementary medicine or integrative medicine or schools of natural medicine scattered about Australasian metropolitan areas. A perusal of the complementary or alternative medicine section of book stores will not only reveal titles of books imported on this topic from the United States and Great Britain, but books specifically designed for the Australian and New Zealand markets, such as *The Encyclopedia of Natural Healing: The Definitive Australian Reference Guide to Treatments for Mind and Body* (Woodham & Peters, 1997) and *The Complete Guide to Integrated Medicine: The Best of Complementary and Conventional Care* (Peters & Woodham, 2000).

I first became interested in the phenomenon of *medical pluralism* – a term that refers to complex societies characterised by a conflation of medical sub-systems which generally compete with one another and sometimes cooperate or collaborate with each other – in the late 1970s and early 1980s while conducting research on religious healers in African American Spiritual churches and delving in the socio-status of osteopathy in the United States and Great Britain (Baer, 1981, 1984a, 1984b, 2001). Adopting a political economy of health and critical medical anthropological perspective (Baer, Singer, & Susser, 2003), I became interested in how patterns of medical pluralism reflect power relations in their respective larger societies. Whereas I had examined medical pluralism in the United States over the course of over two and a half decades and briefly in Britain during the summer of 1983, a visiting position in the School of Archaeology and Anthropology at the Australian National University in Canberra in 2004 gave me the unique opportunity to examine this topic in a two countries that I had previously not as much visited. Whereas most of my research on medical pluralism has occurred in the United States (Baer, 2001, 2004) and some of it in the United Kingdom, in this book I turn my attention to the phenomenal growth of alternative medicine or complementary medicine 'down under', namely in Australia and New Zealand. In January 2006, I immigrated to Australia to assume a continuing position at the University of Melbourne.

Approximately one half of Australians reportedly utilize some form of alternative medicine, with an estimated $AU2.3 million having been spent on it in 2000 (MacLennan, Wilson, & Taylor, 2002). MacLennan et al. (2002) also estimated that Australians spent $AU616 million on alternative consultations in 2000. Indeed, the World Health Organization (2001) estimates that Australians spent approximately AU$ one billion a year on complementary medicine. Finally, Bensoussan, Myers, Wu, and O'Connor (2004) estimated that some 1.9 million naturopathic and Western herbal medicine consultations occurred in Australia in 2003. Despite the 2003 scandal involving Pan Pharmaceuticals, a major manufacturer of natural products in Australia, MacLennan, Myers, and Taylor (2006), based upon a third survey of utilization of complementary medicine in South Australia, extrapolated that Australians spent AU$1.8 billion on complementary medicine in 2004.

Complementary and alternative medicine (CAM) does not appear to be either as popular or legitimised in New Zealand as it is in Australia, but its presence is overtly apparent in everyday social life. The 2002/03 New Zealand Health Survey provides provisional results in terms of the number of New Zealand adults who visited a CAM practitioner at least once during a 12-month period (Ministerial Advisory Committee on Complementary and Alternative Health, 2004:67). This study indicated that 23.4 percent of the respondents (28.1 percent female, 18.4 percent male) had visited a complementary and alternative practitioner. In another survey, of 438 New Zealand adults, 28 percent felt that that alternative therapies offer an equal or better chance of curing cancer than biomedical treatment, 34 percent disagreed with this idea, and 38 percent said that they did not know (Trevena & Reeder, 2005).

Although I found some materials on complementary medicine in the library system of the Australian National University, the National Library of Australia and the library at Southern Cross University proved to be better sources of materials on complementary medicine. In March 2004 I met various practitioners, including naturopaths, at the 5th International Conference of Phytotherapeutics sponsored by the National Herbalists Association of Australia in Canberra. I also had the opportunity to present seminars in the School of Natural and Complementary Medicine at Southern Cross

University on two occasions – July 2004 and again in October 2004. I had the opportunity to interact again with Stephen Myers, the Director of the Australian Centre of Complementary Medicine, and Paul Orrock, the Head of the School of Natural and Complementary Medicine, both of whom I had met at the American Association of Naturopathic Physicians Meeting in August 2002 in Salt Lake City, Utah. Furthermore, I was also able to interact with numerous other staff members, including Sue Evans (a herbalist-naturopath), Tini Grueber (a naturopath-nutritionist), and Ian Howden (a homeopath) and students, particularly Aidre Grant (a PhD student in naturopathic medicine and a macrobiotics instructor) in the school upon those occasions, thus enabling me to gain valuable insights on the socio-political status of naturopathy, Western herbalism, homoeopathy, and complementary medicine in general in Australia. I also had the opportunity to discuss the socio-political status of Australian osteopathy with Rod Harris, an osteopath with offices in Canberra and Moss Vale, New South Wales, on several occasions when he treated me for a back problem and Evan Lallemand, a Canberra-based osteopath who over the past several decades has played a pivotal role in the politics of Australian osteopathy.

In January 2006, I returned to Australia, but this time permanently and assumed a joint position in the Development Studies Program in what was then the School of Anthropology, Geography, and Environmental Studies and the Centre for Health and Society at the University of Melbourne. I have established contacts with several complementary practitioners in the Melbourne area, including several who have been or are presently postgraduate students in the Masters of Social Health program at the University of Melbourne, members of the Victorian Herbalists Association, and academic staff members at the Southern School of Natural Therapies and the Melbourne branch of the Australian College of Natural Medicine. These individuals have enlightened me about the socio-political status of complementary medicine in both the local area and Australia at large. Ironically, some of the students in the postgraduate programs in social health in the Centre of Health and Society at the University of Melbourne are trained naturopaths, including three of whom took my Culture, Health, and Illness subject in semester 1 of 2006. These three students, Cheryl Beale, Rachel Canaway, and Gregg Connolly and I presented a seminar in the Centre of Health and Society on 6 November 2006 titled 'A dialogue between naturopathy and critical medical anthropology: toward a holistic concept of health'. On 21–23 September 2007 I attended the 6th International Conference on Phytotherapeutics in Cancer where I presented a lecture entitled 'The growing legitimation of complementary medicine in Australia: successes and dilemmas'. At the conference I met Dominique Finney, a Queensland naturopath, who invited me to present two talks in the folk medicine stream at the Woodford Folk Festival. I presented a talk titled 'How holistic is complementary medicine?: a critical medical anthropological perspective' on 30 December 2008 and a talk on the growing legitimation of complementary medicine in Australia the following day. On New Year's Day 2009 I had an opportunity to be a participant in a panel discussion on 'medical freedom' with Dominique as well as two other naturopaths, one of whom specialises in homeopathy, two biomedical physicians interested in complementary medicine, a dance therapist, a musician who produces music therapy CDs, and a layperson who writes books about complementary therapies. Last but not least, I am very appreciative of the insights that Vincent di Stefano (2006), an osteopath and naturopath who authored *Holism and Complementary Medicine: Origin and Principles*, has provided me about Australian complementary medicine in our various conversations.

Obviously various institutions and individuals, some of which I have mentioned, have played a role in the fruition of this book. I particularly appreciate comments that Ian Coulter, a medical sociologist based at the University of California at Los Angeles; Evan Willis, a health sociologist at La Trobe University; Kevin White, a health sociologist at the Australian National University; Gary Easthope, a health sociologist at the University of Tasmania; Kevin Dew, a health sociologist at Victoria University of Wellington, and Lesley Cuthbertson, a nurse educator at Flinders University, made on earlier drafts of this book. They, of course, are not responsible for the manner in which I incorporated their comments or failed to do so. I also am grateful to Fran Collyer, a health sociologist at the University of Sydney, who first put me in contact with James Davidson, the publisher of eContent Management P/L and The Australian Sociological Association's *Health Sociology Review*.

Introduction

*I*n the late nineteenth century, on the eve of the formation of Australia and New Zealand as nation-states, the medical systems in these two societies could be best described as pluralistic in the sense that, while regular medicine constituted the predominant medical system, it was not clearly the dominant one in that regular physicians faced competition from a wide array of alternative practitioners. As regular medicine increasingly assumed the guise of being scientific, it evolved into biomedicine and developed a link with corporate and state interests in the early twentieth century in both Australia and New Zealand, as in other capitalist developed societies. Relying upon state support, biomedicine in Australia and New Zealand achieved dominance over alternative medical systems, such as homeopathy, herbal medicine, osteopathy, chiropractic, and naturopathy. Alternative medical systems, however, often do not accept biomedical dominance and often seek to draw upon both support from satisfied patients, as well as strategic elites, in furthering their legitimation. Various social forces, particularly the development of the holistic health movement, served to challenge biomedical dominance in Australia and New Zealand, like elsewhere, beginning in the early 1970s. Indeed, since the early 1970s alternative therapeutic systems, such as chiropractic, osteopathy, Chinese medicine and acupuncture, naturopathy, Western herbalism, homeopathy, and various forms of bodywork, have grown in popularity in Australasia. What started out as a popular health movement has evolved into the professionalized entity that is generally referred to as 'complementary medicine' in Australia and 'complementary and alternative medicine' or 'complementary and alternative health' in New Zealand. In reality, complementary medicine or CAM in both countries encompasses many medical systems and therapies.

Since the 1980s certain heterodox medical systems, particularly chiropractic, osteopathy, acupuncture and Chinese medicine, naturopathy, Western herbalism, and homeopathy, have achieved considerable recognition from the Australian government, either at the federal level or at the state and territorial levels, and the New Zealand government at the national level. The Australian government appears to have gone further than any other Anglophone country in terms of providing public funding for complementary medicine education. Conversely, it has committed a limited amount of funding for complementary medicine research compared to the United States. The New Zealand government also has expressed a growing interest in CAM, but has been much more restrictive in terms of its funding for both complementary medicine education and research.

The rise of biomedicine as the dominant medical system in Australia

As Table 1 below illustrates, since the beginning of the twentieth century, like elsewhere in the world, biomedicine clearly came to dominate rival medical systems in Australia. It formed associations to challenge competition, lobbied the state to ban or at least restrict heterodox practitioners or 'quacks', formed alliances with conservative forces in the corporate sector, and came to dominate research on health-related issues.

Pensabene (1980) examines the rising power of what might be termed 'regular medicine' in the nineteenth century and what might be termed,

Table 1 Medical pluralism in Victoria, 1881*

Medical practitioner	Male	Female	Total
Registered medical physicians	454	–	454
Chemists, druggists and assistants	755	6	761
Dentists	105	2	107
Opticians	22	–	22
Midwives	–	540	540
Unregistered Chinese physicians	35	–	35
Unregistered Indian physicians	1	–	1
Other unregistered physicians, surgeons and assistants	6	–	6
Unregistered aurists and occultists	7	–	7
Unregistered homeopaths	–	1	1
Hydopathists	6	1	7
Herbalist	9	–	9
Medical galvanists	9	–	9
Medical botanists	1	–	1
Medical mesmerists	1	–	1
Chiropodists	4	–	4
Medical magnetists	1	1	2
Medical clairvoyants	–	1	1
Psychopathists	1	–	1
Other irregular practitioners	3	–	3
Total	420	552	1972

*Source: Adapted from table in Pensabene (1980:7) drawing from Victorian State Census of 1881

following medical anthropological terminology, 'biomedicine' in the 20th century in the state of Victoria. He argues that the evolution of these incarnations of conventional medicine followed a similar trajectory in other parts of Australia. Pensabene asserts that,

> [T]he professional status and power of the doctor in the late nineteenth century was low, as evidenced by public questioning of the professional skill and expertise of the registered medical practitioner. Only after 1900 did his professional status improve substantially (Pensabene, 1980:4).

In the late nineteenth century, the Victorian medical system could be best described as a pluralistic one.

While not a heterodox practitioner per se, the chemist, according to Pensabene (1980:8), functioned as both an alternative and complementary practitioner to the regular physician in that he dispensed drugs prescribed by the physician but also frequently offered 'shop-front' medical care based upon the patient's description of his or her symptoms. He prepared many drugs from their chemical bases and had an extensive knowledge of their properties and side effects. 'Unregistered alternative practitioners' constituted the second main alternative to certified medical practitioners and tended to be concentrated in cities and ranged from those who had degrees from foreign regular medical schools, but had not be able to obtain certification in Victoria, to homeopaths to occult practitioners (Pensabene, 1980:8). Despite the fact that the majority of them were self-trained, many used medical titles. John B. Hickson, reportedly the first homeopathic physician in Victoria, practiced in Melbourne during the 1850s (Pensabene, 1980:134). The Melbourne Homeopathic Dispensary was established in 1869 and the Melbourne Homeopathic Hospital was established in 1876 (Pensabene, 1980:137). While a few homeopaths came from Britain, most of them had emigrated from the United States. Like in other countries, Australian homeopathy became divided between the purists who strictly followed Hahnemannian principles and the mixers who incorporated aspects of regular medicine. By the 1920s, all of the honorary medical staff at Melbourne Homeopathic Hospital used allopathic medications. During the nineteenth century, in Victoria and elsewhere in Australia, homeopathy served as a strong rival to regular medicine and received staunch support from various strategic economic, political, and clerical elites in Australian society (Willis, 1989a:58). While the South Australian Branch of the British Medical Association attempted but failed in its effort to forbid its members to professionally interact with homeopathic physicians, the state allowed the 'registration of homeopathic practitioners, thus granting them *de jure* formal medical qualifications' (White, 1999:182).

Prior to 1890, the regular medical profession in Victoria and Australia as a whole consisted primarily of British-trained physicians (Pensabene, 1980:57). According to Richards (1994:25), the 'vast majority' of the '223 medical practitioners who were colonial residents at the time of the formal inauguration of the Queensland branch of the BBA [British Medical Association] in May 1984' had obtain their training in Britain. Of these early Queensland medical practitioners, 83 came from England, 65 from Scotland, 45 from Ireland, and only 20 of them were native-born Australians (Richards, 1994:35).

With the creation of medical schools at the University of Melbourne in 1862, the University of Sydney in 1883, and the University of Adelaide in 1885, Australian-trained regular physicians became more commonplace. The rapid increase in the number of regular physicians during the late nineteenth century and first decade of the twentieth century prompted concern among established regular medical practitioners (Pensabene, 1980:78). Furthermore, in New South Wales and presumably elsewhere in Australia 'there were growing tensions between medical elites (in the main hospital consultants, notably surgeons) and rank and file practitioners' (Lloyd, 1994:22). The creation of specialist colleges beginning in the 1920s contributed to stiff competition for consultancies.

The cost of regular medical education, however, tended to serve as an important factor in the transformation of regular medicine into a high-status occupation. According to Willis,

> Entry to [regular] medicine...required substantial family backing involving the purchase of both a private school and university education. Once qualified there were further costs which heightened this class restrictiveness, such as the cost of setting up in practice. As a result, three quarters of native born doctors who commenced practice during the 1880s were sons of professional men (Willis, 1989a:60).

As regular medicine increasingly assumed the guise of being scientific, it evolved into biomedicine in the early part of the twentieth century and increasingly achieved dominance over heterodox practitioners. Like in the United States, Britain, and other capitalist industrial societies, the germ theory, which downplayed the role of political-economic and social-structural determinants of disease by focusing on biological determinants, appealed to the Australian capitalist class and its political allies situated in the state apparatus. As Willis says (1989a:89), observes various 'business interests, both national and international, were involved in promoting the paradigm of scientific medicine in Victoria'. The Rockefeller Foundation, which had played a key role in the development of biomedicine in the United States, donated 100,000 pounds in the late 1920s for the construction and equipping of clinical laboratories at the University of Sydney (Willis, 1989a:88). In contrast to medical legislation passed prior to 1880, which did little to restrict the practices of heterodox practitioners in Australia, medical legislation passed first in 1908 and then in 1933 ensured the dominance of regular medicine or biomedicine over rival medical systems. Willis asserts that,

> [t]he 1908 Act required a major victory for scientific medicine, ensuring a position of domiance within the health arena. Foreign registration was effectively ended and the supply of doctors more easily regulated...homeopathy and other modes of medicine [such as herbalism] were effectively controlled, indeed the passing of the Act marked the bginning of the end of homeopathy (Willis, 1989a:74).

The 1908 Act also limited the registration of new homeopathic physicians to only one a year (Willis, 1989a:79). Homeopaths had been able to prescribe under the guidelines of the 1886 Poisons Act. Furthermore, homeopathic pharmacy shops operated and even sold homeopathic kits to rural customers (Easthope, 2004:314). The Medical Council in Tasmania during the first decade of the twentieth century included two homeopathic physicians among its nine members (Easthope, 2004:315). Despite biomedical opposition, homeopaths and two homeopathic hospitals managed to function until around 1930. The supply of homeopathic physicians from Britain to Tasmania and presumably other parts of Australia eventually ended because the National Insurance Act of 1911 enabled homeopathic physicians to develop thriving practices in the mother country (Easthope, 2004:315). According to Weir,

> The only homeopathic hospital in Melbourne (now Prince Henry Hospital) became OM [orthodox medicine] as it was difficult to find sufficient homeopaths to fill positions in the hospital. By relaxing the ethical rules about dealing with homeopaths the hospital was able to appoint OM practitioners and gradually the use of homeopathy in the hospital declined until in 1934 the hospital was renamed and no longer represented itself as a homeopathic institution (Weir, 2005:65–66).

Locally-trained biomedical physicians constituted the largest portion of the biomedical profession after 1911 (Pensabene, 1980:57). Over 80 percent of biomedical physicians were Australian-trained by 1933. The Port Phillip Medical Association was established in 1846 and became the Victorian Medical Association (Pensabene, 1980:99). The Medico-Chirurgical Society was established in June 1854. Pensabene (1980:99) delineates three phases in emergence of the 'medical union': (1) 1875–1905 during which a number of competing associations, namely the Medical Society of Victoria, Victorian Branch of the BMA, Medical Defence Association, Melbourne Medical Association, and a small number of country societies; (2) 1905–1925 which witnessed the merger of the various associations into the BMA and MDA; and (3) 1925–1935 during which the bifurcation of Australian biomedicine into general practitioners and specialists occurred with the creation in 1936 of the Australasian College of Surgeons occurred. According to Gillespie (1991:241), by the late 1940s the British Medical Association 'had emerged from disarray to become the model of a united pressure group, single-mindedly pursuing the goal of provide private medicine, subsidized but not controlled by the state'.

Relying upon state support, by the 1930s biomedicine had achieved dominance over other alternative medical systems, such as homeopathy, herbal medicine, osteopathy, chiropractic, and naturopathy, which came to be either excluded or marginalised within the context of the Australian plural medical system (Willis, 1989a:36–91). The biomedical profession in Australia severed its ties with the British Medical Association by forming a separate Australian Medical Association in 1961. Despite the implementation of Medibank in 1972 under the auspices of the Labour government and Medicare in 1984 again under the auspices of the Labour government, the biomedical profession was able to maintain professional autonomy over their work under a constitutional amendment (Belcher, 2002:277). Nevertheless, it is important to note that Australian biomedicine is not a monolithic entity. The implementation of Medibank prompted factionalism within biomedicine due to disagreements over the issue of remuneration. According to Wearing,

> The Doctors Reform Society formed to argue for remuneration through salaries and not on the fee for service basis support by the AMA. This salary argument challenged the privileges and remuneration from voluntary (private) health insurance that covered those able to take out insurance and ensured doctors' high fees could be met (Wearing, 2004:272).

By 1997, AMA membership had declined to less than 60 percent of biomedical physicians in Australia (Wearing, 2004:273).

Nevertheless, in achieving its hegemonic status, Willis (1989a) asserts that Australian biomedicine employed four methods in its efforts to exert dominance over its competitors: (1) subordination that ensured that some health workers, such as nurses and midwives, were placed under the direct authority of biomedical physicians; (2) limitation that legally restricted the occupational domain of certain health workers, particularly dentists, optometrists, podiatrists, and physiotherapists, through biomedical representation on registration boards; (3) exclusion by denying legitimacy to heterodox practitioners, such as chiropractors, osteopaths, naturopaths, herbalists, homeopaths, and acupuncturists, by excluding them from registration, state-supported education and research, and nationalized health coverage; and (4) incorporation of certain medical procedures, such as child delivery, spinal manipulation, and more recently acupuncture, into the scope of biomedical practice.

The rise of biomedicine as the dominant medical system in New Zealand

In contrast to Australia, a country of some 21 million people, complementary medicine has not received nearly as much historical and social scientific attention in New Zealand, understandable given that it has approximately a fifth the population. The 1906 reported that existence of 125 quack 'specialists' (Duke, 2005:11). The Quackery Prevention Act of 1908 proposed the possible regulation of alternative medical systems. Like in Australia, biomedicine historically has had close linkages with the UK. According to Dew,

> During the early period of colonisation, doctors and chemists were the only health workers with distinct occupational status. In the 1870s other occupational groups, such as dentists, opticians, masseurs and public health officials, emerged. Nurses and trained midwives became more numerous in the 1880s. Homeopaths remained within the registered medical profession, but herbalists, hydrotherapists and medical electricians were excluded (Dew, 2003:27).

Statutory regulation of regular medical physicians started early in New Zealand with the New Munster Ordinance of 1849, which provided allopathic practitioners in New Munster, an area south of the Patea River, with a license to practice (Dew, 2003:27). However, the push on the part of different provinces to create their own regulatory legislation weakened efforts on the part of regular physicians for a centralised regulatory system. The Medical Practitioners Act of 1867 guaranteed the dominance of regular medicine at the national level and aimed to undermine homeopathy by including a provision adopted 'British pharmacopoeia as the only prescription source in public hospitals', thereby excluding homeopathy from the hospital system, despite strong backing from wealthy patients of this heterodox medical system (Dew, 2003:28). The high status of homeopathy, however, is evidenced by the fact that the government appointed a homeo-path as an assessor who examined the qualifications of applicants for medical registration. When the government refused to dismiss the appointee, the Medical Board resigned in protest, thus prompting the government to pass the Medical Practitioners Act of 1869, which placed the regulation of phy-sicians in the office of the Registrar-General. Under this system, medical practitioners were only required to submit proof of qualification from an approved medical college which required three years of study.

Finally the passage in 1914 of the Medical Practitioners Act in 1914 strengthened the dominance of the biomedical profession. Medical doctors with less than five years of overseas training were excluded and graduates of the Otago Medical School (est. 1874) became the standard bearer of medi-cal orthodoxy. According to Dew,

> Because it had come under some criticism for not being able to offer its students as much clinical experience as the better overseas schools did, because of the small size of the teaching hospital in Dunedin, the Otago school was prompted to offer a very conservative medical edu-cation in order to avoid further criticisms. That is, any educational experiences that were outside a strict orthodoxy might attract further concern about the educational standards of the Otago Medical School, and therefore they did not find their way on to the local medical cur-riculum (Dew, 2003:30).

According to Davis (1981:109), the New Zealand state played a pivotal role in guaranteeing biomedicine with 'occupational monopoly'.

In contrast to Britain where at least one heterodox medical system, namely homeopathy, enjoyed some semblance of prestige, as evidenced by the existence of an array of homeopathic hospitals, regular medicine or what evolved into biomedicine reigned supreme in New Zealand. As Dew (2003:30) so astutely observes, 'By 1940 the New Zealand medical profession was homogenous, organised and a powerful pressure group, with medical knowledge and education having become much more standardised'.

Despite the quick ascendency of regular medicine or biomedicine in New Zealand, alternative medicine has operated at the fringes of society in the country since the nineteenth century. 'Irregular practitioners' report-edly comprised 20 percent of physicians in the mid-1890s (Dew, 2003:34). Until around 1914, homeopaths and herbalists provided what have become biomedical physicians with their fiercest competition. Belgrave (1985:310) argues that the decline of homoeopathy and herbalism ended any serious challenge to biomedical dominance.

Alternative challenges to biomedical dominance

Alternative medical systems historically have not accepted biomedical dominance passively and have with varying success challenged it through processes of professionalisation and lobbying of strategic elites in the corporate and state sectors. As a result of its perceived contribution to functional health, which is essential for maintaining a productive workforce, entry into the role of health care provider in capitalist societies has historically been viewed as a vehicle for improving one's socio-economic status. When individuals from lower social strata are denied entrance into the dominant medical profession, they sometimes turn to alternative healing groups as a vehicle for pursuing upward social mobility. Professionalised heterodox systems, such as osteopathy, chiropractic, naturopathy, and herbalism, have held out the promise of improved social mobility to numerous lower-middle-class and working-class individuals as well as members of other social categories. In attempting to enter the medical marketplace, as Larkin (1983:5) observes, 'innovatory groups in medical science often commence with low status, particularly through their involvement in activities previously regarded as outside of a physician's or surgeon's role'. As the new medical system grows, it accumulates,

> more and more members who are interested in making a good living
> and in raising their status in the outer world. In the health sphere, this
> means that they become more concerned with obtaining respectable
> (or at least respectable-looking) credentials, providing services that
> more clearly follow the medical model, and eventually even develop-
> ing relationships with the orthodox world (Roth, 1976:40–41).

In a sense, heterodox practitioners generally aspire to enter the petit bourgeoisie. Under corporate or late capitalism, as Szymanski and Goertzel (1979:54) assert, 'the *petit bourgeois* system of production survives primarily in service industry where personal relationships between seller and customers are important'. Many heterodox practitioners have emulated, and continue to emulate, the entrepreneurial, pecuniary practices of the competitive sector of their respective societies. In this capacity, complementary practitioners often range from those who earn a respectable income to those who struggle to make financial ends meet (Andrews & Phillips, 2005).

The drive for professionalisation on the part of heterodox practitioners has historically entailed the following processes: (1) claim of a distinctive body of knowledge and expertise; (2) the creation of organisational structures, including associations, schools, voluntary registries, and codes of ethics; (3) lobbying for statutory recognition in one form or other for preferably full-practice rights or at least limited practice rights; and (4) an effort to establish a monopoly over specific work tasks. Needless to say, the drive for professionalisation is part and parcel of a larger endeavour, namely the drive for legitimacy and closure. According to Willis,

> Legitimacy is a politico-legal process whereby a set of practices is accepted as authoritative and becomes dominant through the political process. The practices [in the case of both biomedicine and alternative medical systems] are a set of diagnostic and therapeutic techniques based upon a paradigm of knowledge, which an occupation utilises in the performance of its services...Legitimacy is not related to a single 'truth' standard, even if such a standard could be decided on the basis of criteria other than those internal to the paradigm itself (Willis, 1989b:260).

Various social forces have developed over the past three decades or so that have served to challenge biomedical dominance in Australia and New Zealand. In the Australian case, according to Germov (2002), these include: (1) the professionalisation strategies of allied health practitioners within the corridors of biomedicine itself; (2) broader notions of health that emphasise prevention and community care; (3) regulatory efforts on the part of the state that aim to cut costs and assess the quality and effectiveness of health care delivery; (4) a decline in the authority enjoyed by biomedicine as a result of media exposés of medical fraud and negligence; (5) '*the increasing popularity of alternative therapies*' (emphasis mine); and (6) the growing concern for patient rights. Examples of the corporatisation of biomedicine include the proliferation of for profit hospitals and one-stop medical centres where physicians are paid a salary or a portion of the fee.

In keeping with Germov's observation about alternative therapies, like in virtually all other countries, heterodox, alternative or complementary medical systems [the latter term has become commonplace in Australia] have become increasingly popular among health consumers since the early 1970s due to increasing dissatisfaction with the bureaucratic, iatrogenic, and high costs of biomedicine. Fogliani and Khoury (2003) argue that Senator Bob Wood's use of the term 'complementary medicine', as opposed to 'alternative medicine' or 'complementary and alternative medicine', when he spoke in his capacity as the Parliamentary Secretary to the Commonwealth Minister of Health at the 1996 Alternative Medicine Summit prompted its usage in Australian health discourse. Complementary medicine in Australia is part and parcel of an international health movement generally referred to as 'complementary and alternative medicine' (CAM). According to Hess (2004:696), '[t]he field of CAM is a complex amalgam of reformers within the medical profession and associated research communities, industries and government bodies, as well as alternative healthcare professions, lay healers and patient-advocacy organizations'.

What started out as the popular holistic health movement in the early 1970s in large part evolved into the professionalised entity generally referred to as CAM or 'integrative medicine'. Alternative medicine generally refers to all medical systems or therapies lying outside the purview of biomedicine that are used instead of it. Complementary medicine refers to medical systems or therapies that used alongside of or as adjuncts to biomedicine. Finally, integrative medicine refers to the effort on the part of conventional physicians to biomedical and CAM therapies, or the collaborative efforts between biomedical practitioners and CAM practitioners in addressing the health care needs of specific patients.

Conceptions of what medical systems or therapies fit within the rubric of complementary and alternative medicine or complementary medicine in the case of Australia vary widely (Drury, 1985; Easthope, 1999:272; Wiesner, 1989). While Pietroni (1992) and Fulder (1993) apparently developed their respective typologies of CAM therapies with the UK primarily in mind, their schemes can be easily transposed to other Anglophone countries, including Australia. Pietroni (1992) delineates CAM systems or therapies into four categories: (1) complete systems, such as homeopathy, naturopathy, osteopathy, herbal medicine, and Traditional Chinese Medicine; (2) diagnostic methods, such as iridology, kinesiology, and hair analysis; (3) therapeutic modalities, such as massage, reflexology, and shiatsu; and (4) self-care approaches, such as meditation, yoga, and dietetics. Fulder (1993) delineates four types of CAM systems or modalities: (1) ethnic medical systems, such as Ayurveda and Traditional Chinese Medicine; (2) manual therapies, such as osteopathy, chiropractic, reflexology, and massage; (3) mind–body therapies, such as hypnotherapy, psychic healing, and Anthroposophical medicine; (4) nature-care therapies, such as naturopathy and hygienic practices; and (5) non-allopathic medicinal systems, such as homoeopathy and herbalism.

The National Centre for Complementary and Alternative Medicine, a division of the US National Institute of Health, defines CAM as 'a group of diverse medical and health care systems, practices, and products that are not presently considered to be part of conventional medicine', which in its view includes biomedical physicians, osteopathic physicians, nurses, and various allied health professionals, such as physical therapists and psychologists (nccam.nih.gov, accessed 18/02/2009). NCCAM recognises for major types of complementary and alternative medicine:

- Whole medical systems which are 'built upon complete systems of theory and practices', such as Ayurveda and Traditional Chinese Medicine.
- Mind–body medicine which 'uses a variety of techniques designed to enhance the mind's capacity to affect bodily function and symptoms', such as prayer, mental healing, art therapy, music therapy, and dance therapy.

- Biologically based practices which 'use substances found in nature, such as herbs, foods, and vitamins'.
- Manipulative and body-based practices which 'are based on and/or movement of one or more parts of the body', such as chiropractic.
- Energy medicine which 'involve the use of energy fields', such as Reiki and Therapeutic Touch.

The New South Wales Department of Health defines 'complementary health' as a 'heterogenous collection of therapeutic substances and techniques based on theory and explanatory mechanisms that are not consistent with the western clinical model of medicine' (NSWHEALTH, 2002:3). It identifies the following types of complementary health practised in Australia: Traditional Chinese Medicine, acupuncture, naturopathy, homoeopathy, Western herbal medicine, Ayurvedic medicine, massage therapy, shiatsu, Reiki, chelation therapy, chiropractic and osteopathy (NSWHEALTH, 2002:4–6). The federal government's Expert Committee on Complementary Medicines in the Health System (2003 – see Appendix B) delineated the classificatory scheme depicted in Table 2 below.

Table 2
Classification of complementary health systems

A. Traditional medicine systems
1. Traditional Chinese Medicine
2. Acupuncture
3. Ayurvedic medicine
4. Kanpo medicine
5. Western herbal medicine

B. Other systems
1. Anthroposophical medicine
2. Homoeopathy
3. Bach and other flower remedies
4. Nutritional medicine
5. Aromatherapy
6. Naturopathy

C. Manipulative therapies
1. Massage therapy
2. Shiatsu
3. Reiki
4. Chiropractic
5. Osteopathy

D. Other therapies
1. Chelation therapy
2. Magnetic field theory

An anthology edited by Terry Robson (2003) entitled *An Introduction to Complementary Medicine* includes chapters on four 'philosophies of healing', namely Ayurveda, Indigenous healing, naturopathic medicine, Traditional Chinese Medicine, and eleven 'healing modalities' – namely acupuncture, aromatherapy, chiropractic, counselling, flower essences, herbal medicine, homeopathy, massage therapy, nutrition, osteopathy, and yoga and meditation – that are currently practised in Australia. In reality, any particular medical system may encompass various therapeutic modalities. For example, naturopathy draws upon spinal manipulation, herbal medicine, homeopathy, massage therapy, nutrition, and more recently Ayurveda, acupuncture, and counselling. CAM or CM therapies generally subscribe to the concept of vitalism – 'that all living organisms are sustained by a vital force that is both different from and greater than physical and chemical forces' (Coulter & Willis, 2004:587).

What has come to be termed 'complementary medicine' in Australia and 'complementary and alternative medicine' in the United States, Canada, and Great Britain as well as New Zealand is an amorphous category that encompasses many medical systems and therapies. As Easthope (2004:311) observes, '[w]hat constitutes CAM changes over time and between countries because CAM can be defined only in relation to the orthodox'. For example, while overviews of CAM or complementary medicine include hypnotherapy in a litany of therapeutic modalities, many biomedical physicians (including psychiatrists), dentists, and clinical psychologists use it in their practices both in the United States and Australia as well as elsewhere. Willis (1989b:60), a medical sociologist who has examined particularly chiropractic and Traditional Chinese Medicine, identifies three major 'complementary modalities' in Australia, namely: (1) chiropractic and osteopathy as manual medical systems that within the Australia scenario have become somewhat intertwined, despite efforts to remain distinctive; (2) 'natural therapies' which encompass a wide array of modalities, such naturopathic, herbal medicine, homeopathy, massage therapy, and even reflexology; and (3) Traditional Chinese Medicine, which encompasses both acupuncture and Chinese herbal medicine.

Most typologies of complementary medicine tend to privilege Western and Asian therapies over Indigenous, folk, and religious therapies and may exclude certain therapeutic systems or therapies. Furthermore, the distinction between conventional medicine and complementary or alternative medicine is a matter of historical circumstances and socio-cultural setting (Frohock, 2002). For example, whereas osteopathy emerged as a distinct alternative medical system in the late nineteenth century in the United

States, in its place of its origin it quickly evolved into osteopathic medicine and surgery or a parallel medical system to biomedicine and can for the most part be included within the rubric of conventional medicine. Conversely, in other Anglophone countries, namely, Canada, Britain, Australia, and New Zealand, osteopathy, like chiropractic, continues to function primarily as a manual medical system and can still be categorized, with some qualifications, as complementary or alternative (Baer, 2004). Parker (2003:1) maintains that the terms 'complementary' and 'alternative' function more or less as 'terms of exclusion that imply lesser status'. He asserts that the aspirations of CAM modalities to be recognised 'will be self-defeating in terms of maintaining an identity that is distinct from orthodox medicine.' (Parker, 2003:1).

Since the 1980s certain heterodox medical systems, particularly chiropractic, osteopathy, acupuncture and Traditional Chinese Medicine, and naturopathy, have achieved considerable recognition from the Australian government, either at the federal level or the state level. The New Zealand government has provided considerable recognition of chiropractic and osteopathy, some recognition of Traditional Chinese Medicine and acupuncture, but only partial recognition of various heterodox medical systems, such as naturopathy, Western herbalism, and homeopathy. Conversely, whereas the Australian government has given little recognition to Indigenous Australian medicine, the New Zealand government, has extended a fair amount of recognition to Maori medicine. Undoubtedly, the fact that Maoris constitute about 9–10 percent of the New Zealand population and have their own political party – the Maori Party – in contrast to Indigenous Australians who constitute about 2.4 percent of the Australian population and lack a political party, accounts for this pattern.

Chapter 1 of this book provides a brief history of alternative medicine in Australia prior to 1970. It includes a discussion of alternative therapeutic systems such as homeopathy, Western herbalism, electrotherapy, massage therapy, osteopathy, and chiropractic. Chapter 2 examines the drive for statutory recognition and public funding for training programs on the part of the chiropractic and osteopathic professions in Australia, both before and after the hearings of the Australian government's Joint Select Committee on Osteopathy, Chiropractic, and Naturopathy during the mid-1970s. It also examines the complex relationship between osteopathy and chiropractic – two competing and sometimes overlapping manual medical systems – in Australia. Chapter 3 discusses the development of naturopathy, acupuncture and Traditional Chinese Medicine, as well as various other complementary or alternative medical systems, such as homoeopathy, bodywork, direct-entry midwifery, religious healing, and folk medicine, in the context of the holistic health movement that diffused to Australia from the United States and probably also Great Britain. This chapter also provides an overview of various studies of complementary medicine utilization in Australia. Chapter 4 discusses various governmental inquiries into complementary medicine since 1977, the drive on the part of acupuncturists and Traditional Chinese Medicine practitioners for statutory registration in the state of Victoria, and the still unsuccessful efforts on the part of natural therapists and other complementary practitioners to achieve statutory registration. Chapter 5 provides an overview of the wide array of private colleges of complementary medicine in Australia and the development of public tertiary institutions offering programs in various complementary therapeutic systems as well as research centres focusing on efficacy studies on complementary therapies. Chapter 6 examines the current niche of complementary medicine, particularly chiropractic, osteopathy, naturopathy and other natural therapies, acupuncture and Traditional Chinese Medicine, within the context of the Australian dominative medical system. Chapter 7 considers the mainstreaming of complementary medicine in Australia as is evidenced by a growing interest in it on the part of biomedical physicians, nurses, and the corporate sector. This chapter also examines the nexus between the natural health products industry and the Australian government, particularly the Therapeutic Goods Administration. Chapter 8 provides and overview of the socio-political status of complementary and alternative medicine in New Zealand, including a discussion of the various medical sub-systems within the New Zealand dominative medical system. Finally, Chapter 9 examines why the Australian and the New Zealand governments have increasingly come to express an interest in complementary and alternative medicine, particularly as part of an effort to promote the concept of wellness among Australians and New Zealanders and to contain public expenditures for health care. This chapter also seeks to assess the future of complementary and alternative medicine in Australia and New Zealand; it considers whether CAM is in danger of being co-opted by biomedicine or whether it contains the potential of providing a meaningful counter-hegemonic challenge to it as well the larger Australian and New Zealand societies. Chapter 10, the concluding chapter, poses the question: how holistic *is* complementary medicine?

Chapter 1

Alternative medicine in Australia to 1970

Introduction

Dyason (1988) maintains that other than homeopaths, Australia had few alternative medical practitioners during the nineteenth century. Conversely, Peter J. Phillips (1978), a popular writer who has an illustrated and jaundiced book on alternative medicine in Australia titled *Kill or Cure*, boldly asserts that regular physicians were greatly outnumbered by the 'unregistered followers of various 'isms', charlatans and montebanks, faith healers and bonesetters, herbalists, medical clairvoyants, abortionists and all the rest'. Unfortunately, while colourful enough, his book contains no citations or references and thus no concrete evidence that alternative practitioners overshadowed the regular ones. Conversely, there is evidence that indicates that at least by the late nineteenth century, Australia had come to provide a refuge for an array of alternative practitioners. These included phrenologists, herbalists, hydropaths, lay midwives, spiritual healers, and purveyors of home remedies and patents medicines (Martyr, 2002:63–124). An 1891 census of 110 'irregular medical practitioners' listed 50 males and six females under the broad rubric of 'medical botanist, clairvoyant, galvanist, herbalist, mesmerist, psychopathist' alone (Martyr, 2002:188). Whereas the 1921 census listed 3959 'regular' medical practitioners, it listed 412 'irregular' practitioners (Martyr, 2002:198). Also, many homeopaths had training in regular medicine and at least some regular physicians became practitioners of hydropathy (Phillips, 1978:59). Like today, the boundaries between conventional medicine and unconventional medicine were fluid during nineteenth century and early twentieth century Australia.

Table 3 depicts the number of alternative practitioners in four Australian states, namely New South Wales, Victoria, Queensland, and Western Australia, in 1924 and 1940, respectively (Martyr, 2002:243).

The development of homeopathy and herbalism in Australia

Like in Britain and North America, homeopathic physicians, particularly if they were registered medical practitioners, enjoyed relatively high status in nineteenth-century Australia and were represented by the Homoeopathic

Table 3
Alternative
practitioners in
4 states: Qld,
WA, NSW,
Victoria*

	1924	1940
Herbalists	172	168
Osteopaths	5	20
Chiropractors	4	29
Health food stores	11	49

*Source: PO directories; Adapted from Martyr (2002:242–2550)

Medical Society of Victoria (McGregor, 2000:15). Tasmania passed the first Medical Act – a piece of legislation that permitted both regular and homoeopathic practitioners and pharmacists to prescribe and sell drugs – in the British Empire in 1837 (Easthope, 2004:314). Although the Medical and Pharmacy Act of 1908 theoretically permitted regular physicians to exclude homoeopaths, the Medical Council in Tasmania included two homoeopaths, Dr. Benjafield and Mr. Gould, who 'were major figures in community, sitting on the boards of many charitable enterprises and, particularly in the case of Dr. Benjafield, running several profitable businesses (Easthope, 2004:315). Indeed, some viewed homeopathy as more than a mere alternative to regular medicine but as a vehicle for reforming it (Martyr, 2002:81). In contrast to the United States and Britain, homeopathic physicians, despite a few exceptions, were by and large not admitted into regular medical or biomedical societies in Australia, thus prompting overseas-trained homeopaths to return home (Martyr, 2002:240–241).

Although homeopaths were not admitted into regular medical societies in New South Wales, they managed for a period of time to operate a hospital in Sydney (Martyr, 2002:241). The Melbourne Homeopathic Dispensary (est. 1869) evolved into a hospital in 1876 and flourished as such until the 1920s, when it became the biomedically-oriented Prince Henry's Hospital. It reportedly was treating over 14,000 patients a year by 1915. Elsewhere, the Adelaide Homoeopathic Dispensary was established in the late 1860s (Martyr, 2002:80). The homeopathic hospitals in Melbourne and Hobart were absorbed into biomedical hospitals by the 1940s (Templeton, 1969:147–157). The last homeopathic physician retired from his practice at the Sydney Homoeopathic Hospital in 1941, thus spelling the demise of the facility a few years later (Martyr, 2002:241).

Households and herbalists employed native and exotic plants for medicinal purposes during the nineteenth century in Australia. The Australasian Union of Herbalists was in existence by the 1890s (McGregor, 2000:14). According to Martyr (2002:245), '[t]he Australian Herbalists' Association... was active in the 1920s, particularly in lobbying against restrictive legislation and for the regulation of the herbalism industry'. Western herbalists numbered 42 in Melbourne by 1925 but slowly contracted in numbers afterwards. Some herbalists published books – Matthew Robinson – *The Australian Botanic Guide* and P. Rasmussen – *The Natural Doctor* (1891). Fifty Chinese practitioners reportedly were practising in the Victorian goldfield towns in 1867. Most of them focused on herbalism but they did some acupuncture as well (McGregor, 2000:14). Twenty to fifty Chinese herbalists reportedly were practicing in Victoria, including in Melbourne's Chinatown, between 1870 and the 1930s. Chinese herbalists obtained their training in various ways, including apprenticeships, training in overseas colleges prior to emigrating, and correspondence school courses (Bentley, 2005:41).

The Pharmacy Board in Victoria attempted to create anti-herbalist legislation in 1925, especially after having learned that a group of herbalists were pushing for statutory registration (Bentley, 2005:44). The Australian Herbalist Association, which had some Chinese members, buttressed its opposition to the proposed legislation with a petition containing some 6000 signatures, including those of upper-middle class intellectuals. The Pharmacy Board agreed to a compromise under which AHA members would have been allowed to continue to practice but Stanley Argyle, the legislator who had submitted the bill, refused to accept the compromise, resulting in the withdrawal of the bill. In time, however, on-going opposition from both organized biomedicine and pharmacy led to the decline membership of the AHA which eventually merged with the National Herbalists Association of Australia (NHAA) in the 1940s (Bentley, 2005:46).

The development of electrotherapy and massage in Australia

What constitutes conventional, regular, or orthodox medicine as opposed to unconventional, irregular, unorthodox, heterodox, or alternative medicine varies considerably both historically and cross-culturally. According to Martyr (n.d.), electrotherapy and massage constituted two treatment modalities that were situated at the interstices of regular medicine and alternative medicine in Australia during the late nineteenth century and into the early twentieth century. Howard Freeman, a transplanted American who claimed to be a Professor of Medical Electricity, operated the Freeman and Wallace Electro-Medical and Surgical Institute in Sydney and gave his establishment an aura of respectability by employing Richard Wallace, a Scottish regular physician (Phillips, 1978:37–40). Some regular practitioners adopted electrotherapy, a form of physical therapy that attempts to stimulate damaged muscles by stimulating the blood circulation through the application of galvanic or faradic currents, to relieve pain and in minor operations such as the removal of ulcers and cysts. As regular practitioners began to discard it, alternative practitioners as well as massage therapists incorporated it into their regimens of treatment.

Massage, an ancient art, became a component in the general trend within British regular medicine toward 'physical culture' and began to be cited in Australian regular medical journals during the 1890s (Martyr, n.d.:5). In part because it is a time-consuming endeavour, regular or biomedical physicians began to pass it onto specialists in massage therapy who worked under their supervision. Alfred Peters (1871–1944), who reportedly was one of the first masseurs in Australia, established a clinic in 1888 in Melbourne shortly after emigrating from England (Bentley, 2000:13–14). He claimed to have introduced massage into the Melbourne Hospital and treated various high-level politicians, cricketers and other celebrities. Peters and other masseurs established the Australasian Massage Association in 1907. According to Bentley,

> Integral to their professional identity was a close association with the medical profession, and an adherence to the precepts of modern medical science. To cement this relationship the association included in its code of ethics the prohibition of treating patients without a doctor's referral (Bentley, 2000:15).

Whereas in 1891, there were five massage therapists in New South Wales and eleven in Victoria, by 1905 there were two in Queensland, 35 in New South Wales, 37 in Victoria, eight in Western Australia, and one in South Australia (Martyr, n.d.:6). Massage as a free-standing practice went into decline after World War I. Massage therapists obtained state registration in Victoria in 1922, Queensland in 1928, South Australia and New South Wales in 1945 (Bentley, 2000:15) and created a niche as an adjunct to rehabilitation then changed their name to 'physiotherapists' in 1940. The Australasian Massage Association renamed itself the Australian Physiotherapy Association in 1942 (Martyr, 2002:236).

The development of osteopathy in Australia

Osteopathy was founded in the 1860s by Andrew Taylor Still (1828–1917), an American regular physician and a dabbler in mesmerism and Spiritualism, in response to what he perceived to be the excesses of regular medicine (Trowbridge, 1991). He became disenchanted with regular medicine when it failed to prevent the death of three of his children from meningitis. Based upon detailed anatomical investigations, Still concluded that many, if not all, diseases are caused by faulty articulations or 'lesions' in various parts of the musculoskeletal system. Such dislocations produce disordered nerve connections that in turn impair the proper circulation of the blood and other body fluids. In his private practice, Still began to rely more and more upon manipulation as a form of therapy. He strongly opposed the use of drugs, vaccines, serums, and modalities such as electrotherapy, radiology, and hydrotherapy. In essence, Still synthesized some of the major components of magnetic healing and bonesetting into a unified medical system. He diligently worked as an itinerant physician with Kirksville, Missouri, as his base of operations. Along with William Smith, a graduate of the University of Edinburgh Medical School, Still established the American School of Osteopathy in Kirksville in September 1892.

Osteopathy appealed to thousands of ordinary rural and small-town people in the United States, particularly those who were suffering from chronic spinal or joint ailments. The creation of an additional 17 osteopathic schools between 1895 and 1900 offered many individuals of humble origins the hope of become medical practitioners (Albrecht & Levy, 1982:74). Despite Still's eschewal of drugs and surgery except in extreme circumstances, American osteopathy began to incorporate more and more aspects of regular medicine or biomedicine. Gradually, American osteopaths came to utilize surgery, drugs, vaccines, and antibiotics and became osteopathic physicians and surgeons. By the 1930s, osteopathic medicine in the United States essentially had become a parallel medical system to biomedicine with an emphasis on general practice and in which manipulative therapy functioned for the most part as an adjunct. By the early 1970s, osteopathic physicians had attained full practice rights in all fifty states and the District of Columbia.

Osteopathy also diffused to various other countries, particularly Anglophone countries such as Canada, the United Kingdom, Australia, and New Zealand, where it remained primarily a manual medical system. In Britain, as naturopathy, or nature cure, lost some of its appeal due to the advent of 'wonder drugs', some naturopaths turned to osteopathy (Baer, 1984a). In contrast to various other countries, the development of osteopathy has been intertwined with that of chiropractic in Australia. Willis (1991:60) maintains that most osteopaths in Australia tended to come from Britain rather than the United States. Conversely, Hawkins and O'Neill (1990:19) maintain that Edgar Culley and Florence McGeorge, graduates of the American School of Osteopathy in 1900, were the first osteopaths to practice in Australia. Culley was listed as a 'Doctor of Osteopathy' in the 1909 Directory of Victoria that listed five osteopaths in 1911, two in 1918, four in 1923, eight in 1928, and thirteen in 1936 (Hawkins & O'Neill, 1990:20–21). McGeorge practised in Melbourne between 1913 and 1916, but settled in Nelson, New Zealand. Charles Farnum established an osteopathic practice in Adelaide in 1935 (Hawkins & O'Neill, 1990:21). Warren Judd was the first overseas trained osteopath to practice in New South Wales.

Osteopaths in Victoria managed to achieve inclusion under the 1922 Massage Registration Act. Various private colleges offered courses in osteopathy along with ones on exercise, herbal medicine, nutrition, and massage therapy and often taught osteopathy and chiropractic together (O'Neill, 1994a:45). Students were able to obtain certification in chiropractic, osteopathy, and naturopathy. Alistair McGowan, David Evans, and Leon Van Straten established the Australian Osteopathic Association in 1941, but the organization did not incorporate until 1955 (Hawkins & O'Neill, 1990:22). As opposed to McGowan and Evans, Straten was a graduate of the British School of Osteopathy (est. 1917). In 1956 Jiri Benes became the second BSO graduate to establish a practice in Australia, namely in Melbourne (Hawkins & O'Neill, 1990:22).

Osteopaths in Australia occasionally were prosecuted for calling themselves 'Doctor', even if they had earned a 'Doctor of Osteopathy' from a US osteopathic college. They were excluded from hospital privileges and access to biomedical support services (Hawkins & O'Neill, 1990:23). In contrast to their American counterparts who managed to obtain full practice rights in most states by the late 1950s and in all states and the District of Columbia by the early 1970s, Australian osteopaths were by and large limited to osteopathic manipulation therapy and massage. Hawkins and O'Neill (1990:26) report that as of 1990, 'no more than 60 overseas trained osteopaths have ever practised in Australia'. Locally-trained osteopaths obtained their training either through apprenticeships or instruction at various schools, some of which taught only osteopathy and others which offered diplomas in both chiropractic and osteopathy and yet others which taught an array of natural therapies, including manipulation (Hawkins & O'Neill, 1990:26). In time the locally-trained osteopaths became spread far and wide and more numerous than the overseas-trained osteopaths and were far more likely to combine osteopathy and chiropractic along with other natural therapies (Hawkins & O'Neill, 1990:26–27). F.G. Roberts (1892–1976), who was also a key player in the development of Australian chiropractic and naturopathy, was a pivotal figure in the development of Australian osteopathy. He was listed as osteopath in Directory of Victoria between 1943 and 1947 and had clinics in all states.

A schism existed between overseas graduates and local graduates (Hawkins & O'Neill, 1990:27). Some osteopaths transformed themselves into chiropractors with the creation of the United Chiropractors'

Association in 1961 (Hawkins & O'Neill, 1990:27). Roberts established the Chiropractic and Osteopathic College of Australasia in 1959 (www.coca. com.au/history.htm). In the mid 1960s, this institution dropped the designation 'osteopathic' from its name. Conversely, some practitioners insisted upon remaining osteopaths and formed the United Osteopathic Physicians Guild (O'Neill, 1994a:45). The Australian Chiropractors' Association and the Australian Osteopathic Association (est. 1955 in Victoria) discussed the establishment of a joint organization in the 1960s but remained separate organizations (Hawkins & O'Neill, 1990:35). Indeed, some Australian practitioners attempted to institutionalise a merger of chiropractic and osteopathy as evidenced by names of two professional bodies, namely the Australian Chiropractors, Osteopaths, and Naturopathic Physicians Association and a group called the Chiropractic and Osteopathic Incorporated (Webb Report, 1977:261). Another example of the blending of osteopathy and chiropractic was Wallace C. Brown, DO, DC, ND, who graduated from the Sydney College of Osteopathy in 1961, from the Indiana Chiropractic College in 1963 and was the Foundation President of the Australian Association of Registered Osteopaths (Osteopathy House, n.d.:1). The Victorian Society of Specialist Osteopaths formed in February 1975 (Committee of Inquiry, 1977:267).

James Doyle, an immigrant from England who practiced both chiropractic and osteopathy, established Pax College of Osteopathy in Ballarat in 1933 that was absorbed by Sydney College of Osteopathy in 1970 (Hawkins & O'Neill, 1990:29). A.K. Kaufman established the Sydney College of Osteopathy at Eastwood in 1959 (Osteopathy House, n.d.:3). He had studied at the London School of Natural Therapeutics where he earned a Diploma of Osteopathy and returned to Australia in 1946 (Hawkins & O'Neill, 1990:28). The Sydney College of Osteopathy was renamed the Sydney College of Osteopathy and Chiropractic in 1972 and incorporated simply as the Sydney College of Chiropractic in 1977, but continued to offer diplomas in both chiropractic and osteopathy. This institution was taken over by the Academy of Natural Healing in 1969 without the approval of its Principal Wallace Brown who established the New South Wales College of Osteopathy in 1971 that also offered courses in naturopathy and chiropractic. Evan Lallemand and Bryon Lambert formed the Windsor College of Applied Osteopathy in 1981. International Colleges of Osteopathy was incorporated in 1981 and absorbed both the Windsor College and New South Wales College of Osteopathy (Hawkins & O'Neill, 1990:30). The Chiropractic, Osteopathic and Naturopathic College of South Australia was established in 1963 but became Chiropractic and Osteopathic College of South Australia (Hawkins & O'Neill, 1990:31).

The development of chiropractic in Australia

Like osteopathy, chiropractic blended together elements from various healing and metaphysical systems. Daniel David Palmer, the founder of chiropractic, had experience with Spiritualism, mesmerism, and other esoteric
philosophies. He opened a magnetic healing office in Burlington, Iowa, and
later in Davenport, Iowa. He administered his first 'spinal adjustment' in
Davenport in September 1895, when he cured an African American janitor
of a 17-year deafness. Palmer argued that disease emanates from 'subluxations' or spinal misalignments. These subluxations result in interference
with neural transmission, which in turn triggers dysfunctions in the internal organs. Spinal adjustment restores the normal 'nerve force', and health
ensues. Palmer began to offer instruction at the Palmer Infirmary and
Chiropractic Institute in 1898.

Given the early rivalry between osteopathy and chiropractic as emerging
manual medical systems, it is not surprising that many osteopaths asserted
that chiropractic was a bastardised version of osteopathy. Chiropractors
vehemently objected, and Palmer himself wryly stated in *The Chiropractor's
Adjustor* (1910) that he was 'more than pleased to know that our cousins, the
osteopaths, are adopting chiropractic methods and advancing along scientific
and philosophical lines' (quoted in Gibbons, 1980:13). There is some evidence that indicates that Palmer had received treatments from Still and that
Palmer had learned manipulative techniques from another osteopath (Baer,
1987:178). In contrast to American osteopathy, spinal adjustment remained
an important therapeutic modality within chiropractic both in the United
States and in other parts of the world to which it diffused. The development
of chiropractic in the United States and elsewhere was particularly shaped
by the internecine battles between the 'straights' and 'mixers' – those who
wished to focus on spinal adjustment as a central modality and those who
wished to incorporate many other modalities from particularly naturopathy
(eg, physiotherapy, hydrotherapy, electrotherapy, colonic irrigation, dietetics, exercise, and vitamin therapy). Because of its extreme eclecticism,
naturopathy provided chiropractic mixers with a ready source from which
to add a wide variety of techniques to their own treatment regimen. Despite
its initial effort to function as a form of drugless general practice, chiropractic in both its straight and mixer forms both in the United States and other
countries, such as Canada, Britain, Australia, and New Zealand, by and large
functions as a musculoskeletal specialty.

Willis (1989a:170–191) delineates four periods in the development of
Australian chiropractic: (1) the establishment period (1918–1953) in which
a group of chiropractors emerged in Victoria from the practice of osteopaths
trained in the UK and US-trained chiropractors and the establishment of

various chiropractic associations; (2) the period of expansion (1954–1961) which witnessed a considerable increase in the number of chiropractors trained both in Australia and overseas; (3) the period of agitation (1961–1973) which resulted in the passage of the Western Australian Chiropractors' Act in 1964 and the inclusion of chiropractic under private health insurance plans; and (4) the period of legitimation that began a federal Parliamentary committee report in 1977 which recommended registration for both chiropractors and osteopaths, although not naturopaths and homeopaths. I present a brief discussion of the first three of these periods and incorporate details of the fourth phase in the following chapter.

The establishment period (1918–1953)

Winter (1975:1) maintains that Harold Williams was probably the first chiropractor to practice in Australia upon his arrival after World War I, and Helen Mackenzie, the first female chiropractor in Australia, opened a practice in Sydney in the early 1920s. Willis (1989a:171–172) states that the 'locally trained group of chiropractic practitioners in Victoria evolved from the practice of osteopathy, derived not so much from the United States but indirectly via Great Britain.' According to Peters and Peters,

> The first evidence of an association of chiropractors in Australasia was in New Zealand in 1920. Its president, J.A. Scott, who was also a lawyer, travelled to Australia in 1927 to establish the Australian and New Zealand Chiropractors' Association. Its president, J.A. Scott, who was also a lawyer, travelled to Australia in 1927 to establish the Australian and New Zealand Chiropractors' Association. The difficulties imposed by distance and the small number of members, however, meant its existence could not be sustained (Peters & Peters, 1986:184).

The overlap between chiropractic and both osteopathy and naturopathy was exemplified by the existence of the Australian Chiropractors, Osteopaths and Naturopathic Physicians' Association (est. 1936) (McAllister, 1976). Fredrick George Roberts was a therapeutic eclectic who played a leading role not only in the development of Australian chiropractic but also osteopathy and naturopathy (Willis, 1989a:172). He had studied at the London School of Natural Therapies and returned to Australia in 1914 where he became a 'large presence in alternative medicine, as teacher and publicist, proprietor of clinics, health food shops and rest homes in capital cities and large towns throughout Australia' (Hawkins & O'Neill, 1990:27). He assumed a leading role in the United Practitioners Association and also established the Melbourne Health Academy in 1940, which became the British and Australian Institute of Naturopathy and later the Chiropractic and

Osteopathy College of Australasia in 1959. The Ward Committee Report (1976:6) describes Roberts as 'obviously a man with a flair for adopting fashion in the healing arts' who 'had little difficulty in using various methods of healing which captured the imagination of supporters of drugless therapies in various forms for more than fifty years'.

Chiropractors who had obtained training in the United States regarded themselves as the superior to locally-trained practitioners to whom they referred to as 'pseudos' (Campbell, Dillon, & Polus, 1982:21). J.A. Scott, a New Zealand chiropractor, visited Australia in 1927 where he established the Australian and New Zealand Chiropractors Association (Portelli, 1985:14). The Australian Chiropractors' Association (ACA) was created in 1938 as a staunch proponent of straight chiropractic and distanced itself from various local chiropractic schools that sprung up (O'Neill, 1994a:47; Sweaney, 1989). In time the ACA came to tolerate the presence of mixers within its ranks but it pursued registration only for graduates of North American chiropractic colleges. It reportedly has 53 members by 1959, at least one quarter of whom were North Americans who had established practices in Australia (Campbell et al., 1982:21). The Chiropractic Association of Victoria formed as a schism from the ACA in 1942 over the latter's rejection of application for membership on the part of R. Herzog who had advertised himself as an osteopath (Campbell et al., 1982:220).

The period of expansion (1954–1961)

According to Willis (1989a:174), '[d]uring this period the number of chiropractors both locally and foreign trained increased considerably' and the struggling profession began to campaign for statutory registration and rebates for their services from private insurance carriers. The Radioactive Substances Act passed by the Australian government in 1957 required chiropractors to obtain a license to use x-rays for diagnostic reasons (Peters & Peters, 1986:173). While the Medical Practitioners Act of 1956 exempted chiropractors from provisions relating to other 'unregistered practitioners', this stipulation 'resulted in a groundswell of naturopaths, osteopaths, masseurs, herbalists and other fringe practitioners, who now started to call themselves chiropractors, and within a few years a multitude of training institutions sprang up incorporating somehow the name of chiropractic in the title' (Peters & Peters, 1986:173).

The Chiropractic and Osteopathic College of Australasia operated schools in Sydney and Melbourne. Other Australian chiropractic schools included Chiropractic and Osteopathic College of South Australia in Adelaide, the Australian College of Chiropractic in Melbourne, and Sydney

College of Chiropractic (McAllister, 1976). The United Chiropractors' Association of Australasia formed in 1961 and reportedly constituted a straight organization that supported the Chiropractic College of Australasia in South Melbourne (Ward Committee, 1976:8). The Sydney College of Chiropractic (est. 1959) became associated with the UCA (Campbell, Dillon, & Herzog, 1982:26). The Chiropractors Association of Victoria (CAV) pushed for statutory registration of US-trained chiropractors (Willis, 1989a:175). At a meeting in Sydney on 11–12 November, 1961, the ACA and the CAV merged to form the ACA proper and declared its intention to add branches in Queensland, South Australia, and Western Australia to the existing branch in Victoria (Australian Chiropractors' Association (Victoria) 1961). In 1965 ACA directory listed 36 members 36 members in Victoria, twelve in New South Wales, five in South Australia, two in Tasmania, two in Queensland, and one in Western Australia (Australian Chiropractors' Association (Victorian Branch) 1965).

The period of agitation (1961–1973)

During this period, various governmental committees began to investigate for the purpose of possible statutory recognition (Willis, 1989a:177). Chiropractors finally achieved statutory registration in Western Australia in 1964 but faced opposition from both the Australian Medical Association and the Australian Physiotherapy Association in other states (Bentley, 2000:13). Roberts led a delegation to Victorian Minister of Health seeking chiropractic legislation in 1964 (Hawkins & O'Neill, 1990:28). The United Chiropractors Association of Australasia, primarily a straight body, formed in 1961 as a rival of the ACA and consisted largely of graduates from the Chiropractic College of Australasia in Melbourne (Devereux, 1998:69; Willis, 1989a:179). The Southern Australian Chiropractic Association was established in 1963 and functioned as an affiliate of the South Pacific Federation of Natural Therapeutics and later the South Pacific Council for Natural Therapies (Committee of Inquiry, 1977:264). The Australian Association of Chiropractors, a mixer organization, was established in 1965 and consisted primarily of graduates of the Sydney College of Chiropractic (Committee of Inquiry, 1977:261). Various osteopathic colleges reportedly transformed themselves into chiropractic colleges in the mid- and late 1960s (Campbell et al., 1982:23). In 1972 the Australian and New Zealand Chirorpactors' Associations created the Australasian Committee on Chiropractic Education in order to create a standard of chiropractic education on part with North American chiropractic institutions (Peters & Peters, 1986:183).

Mixers established the Australian Chiropractors, Osteopaths and Naturopathic Physicians Association. Initially it constituted an organization consisting of 'Victorian graduates of one of the local colleges but extended its cover to other Australian-trained practitioners through various amalgamations' (O'Neill, 1994a:48–49). The CAV became the Victorian Branch of ACA in 1961, which expelled some members who allegedly engaged in false advertising (Willis, 1989a:179). The expellees in turn formed the Victorian Society of Chiropractors. The Committee for the Registration of Chiropractors was established in July 1970 as a patient advocacy group pressing for the registration of chiropractors (Peters & Peters, 1986:173). The UCAA, the strongest of the chiropractic groups consisting of locally-trained chiropractors, in 1975 absorbed the Australian Association of Chiropractors, the Australian Federation of Chiropractors, the Chiropractic Association of Queensland, and the Chiropractic Institute Inc. of South Australia (Committee of Inquiry, 1977:265).

This period was also one in which various osteopaths and naturopaths continued to redefine themselves as chiropractors for various legal reasons, including exemptions in New South Wales from the Medical Act. A manifestation of this process is reflected in the fact that the Sydney College of Osteopathy (est. 1959) changed its name initially to the Sydney College of Chiropractic and Osteopathy and then simply to the Sydney College of Chiropractic (Bolton, 1986:15).

The development of naturopathy and natural therapies in Australia

While some naturopaths trace their practice back to Hippocrates and the medical system of ancient Egypt, the more immediate root of modern naturopathy is the tradition of health spas, which were widespread in central Europe in the eighteenth and nineteenth centuries. Naturopathy initially assumed the guise of 'nature cure' in Britain and *Heilpraktik* in Germany. In the United States, Benedict Lust (1872–1945), a German immigrant, purchased the term *naturopathy* from the hydropath John Scheel, who coined the term in 1895 to describe his medical system (Pizzorno, 1996:165). He became the father of American naturopathy as a result of having established the American School of Naturopathy in New York City in 1901 and the Naturopathic Society of America in 1902.

Australian naturopathy appears to have drawn from both British and American naturopathy and became intricately intertwined, as was noted earlier, with both osteopathy and chiropractic. Like in other countries, naturopaths or natural therapists functions as the ultimate therapeutic eclectics.

They regard disease as a response to bodily toxins and imbalances in a person's social, psychic, and spiritual environment: germs are not the cause of disease per se but rather are parasites that take advantage of the body when it is in a weakened state. Because they believe that the healing power of nature, the *vis mediatrix naturae*, can restore one to health, naturopaths emphasize preventive health, education, and client responsibility. In the past, many naturopaths relied heavily on water treatments, colonic irrigation, dietetics, fasting, and exercise. While some naturopaths continue to advocate these modalities, others today draw upon homoeopathy, spinal manipulation, herbal medicine, vitamin therapy, acupuncture and Chinese medicine, and even Ayurveda. According to Bloomfield (1983:116), 'naturopathy for some people means *all* the forms of non-allopathic medicine which depend on 'natural' remedies and treatments'.

Ward (1975:25) reported that naturopaths in Victoria relied upon osteopathy, chiropractic, homeopathy, electrotherapy, hydrotherapy, diet, herbal medicine, iridology, and 'celloids' that were described by Jacka as 'a specialized system of colloidal mineral salts specially prepared… by Blackmore Laboratories'. The development of Australian naturopathy can be divided into three periods: (1) its emergence during the 1920s, 1930s, and 1940s; (2) a holding period between the 1950s and early 1970s; and (3) its explosion from the late 1970s to the present time. In this chapter I discuss the first two periods and discuss the third phase in chapter 3.

Early naturopaths in Australia obtained their training either through apprenticeships, self-education, and overseas training. McCabe (2005:118) maintains that the first naturopathic course of study in Australia was conducted by the by the British and Australian Institute of Naturopathy during 1940s. According to Evans,

> In common with overseas practice, successful practitioners dedicated a percentage of time training other interested persons, both as an altruistic and a commercial venture. Claud Beale, a naturopath practicing in suburb Brisbane, Queensland, in 1914 is reputed, for example, to have trained early figures Maurice Blackmore and Frank Roberts, although it is suggested that he probably did little more than provide both with certificates of training which were common purchased at that time (Evans, 2000b:236).

Frederick. G. Roberts, a native of Hobart, obtained training at the London School of Natural Therapies (Jacka, 1998:8). In 1929 he advertised himself as both a naturopath and an osteopath and established the Roberts' Naturopathic Institute (a rest home) and a company manufacturing herbal products and nutritional supplements in Melbourne (McGregor, 2000:16).

He also created clinics in Ballarat, Geelong, Newcastle, Brisbane, Ipswich, Toowoomba, Maryborough, Bundaberg, Mackay, Adelaide, Perth, and Freemantle; and played a significant role in United Practitioners Association of Australasia. Roberts also established Health Academy in South Yarra which became in 1959 the Chiropractic and Osteopathy College of Australia and yet later simply became the Chiropractic College of Australasia. This institution was absorbed by the Phillip Institute of TAFE in 1978 and later became part of the Royal Melbourne Institute of Technology (McGregor, 2000:16).

Maurice Blackmore, a graduate of the British Naturopathic College, immigrated to Australia in 1923, opened the first health store in Brisbane in 1934, and went on to run the Victorian Branch College of the National Association of Naturopaths, Osteopaths and Chiropractors. He created a laboratory for the manufacture of minerals and vitamins. The overlap between naturopathy and osteopathy and chiropractic was exemplified by the creation in 1936 of the Australian Chiropractors, Osteopaths and Naturopathic Physicians Association (Committee of Inquiry, 1977:261). This body renamed itself the Australian Physicians' Association in 1955 but reverted to its original name in 1970. Its New South Wales branch became the Australian Naturopathic Physicians Association.

From 1942 to 1945, William Pruss (2006:32) reports that he obtained naturopathic training, which included massage, hydrotherapy, and dietetics, at the Sydney School of Naturopathy which was operated by William Roberts, the brother of Frederick G. Roberts. He obtained clinical training at the Melbourne Institute Naturopathy and after working in various clinical settings, established his own clinic in Sydney in 1949.

Percy Alf Jacka became a naturopath by reading books on natural therapies, taking a correspondence course from London, and undergoing an apprenticeship under Cyril Flowers (Jacka, 1998:4). He opened a naturopathic clinic in East Melbourne and reportedly between the 1950s and 1970s 'had the largest naturopathic practice in Victoria and possibly within the whole of Australia' (McGregor, 2000:16). He earned a Diploma of Electrical Engineering from the Gordon Institute of Technology and completed a correspondence course with the British Naturopathic College (Ward, 1975:7). He served as the President of the Victorian branch of the National Association of Naturopaths, Osteopaths and Chiropractors. Jacka authored *Naturopathy – Natural Healing* in which he wrote that 'Naturopathy postulates that there is a Divine Creator, and that there are certain fundamental natural or Divine laws, the contravention of which creates ill-health' (quoted in Ward, 1975:25).

In 1961 Jacka was persuaded by Blackmore to assume leadership of Victorian School of the National Association of Naturopaths, Osteopaths and Chiropractors that became the Southern School of Naturopathy and still later the Southern School of Natural Therapies (Jacka, 1998:22). Alf along with his wife Judy played pivotal roles in the evolution of the college into a major centre of naturopathy or natural therapies. Jacka (1998) had trained as a nurse and developed interests in Theosophy as well as healing, theology, metaphysics, astrology, and philosophy in general. She completed her studies at the college in 1971, started a small practice in Kew and assumed directorship of the college in early 1972. In the early 1970s, students attended classes three nights a week and on Saturday mornings, earned 1400 hours of theoretical work over the course and also did 1500 hours of clinical work over the course of three years (Taylor, 1973). Students pursuing an additional year of study consisting of about 600 theory hours and 1000 clinical hours could earn a diploma in chiropractic.

Many private naturopathic colleges and new naturopathic or natural therapies associations were established during the 1960s and 1970s and added to the list of those that had been created earlier (Evans, 2000b; Martyr, 2002:272–277). Apparently tensions between Alf Jacka and the association prompted him and his partner to re-establish the school as an independent institution (Canaway, 2007:50). The college initially operated out of the naturopathic clinic operated by Alf and Judy Jacka [They were married in 1976], moved to a later clinic location in Kew in early 1972, still another clinic location in Hawthorn, onto Curtin House on Swanston Street, and finally in 1978 to its present location on Victoria Street in Fitzroy where it eventually was renamed the Southern School of Natural Therapies (Jacka, 1998).

The College of Naturopathic Sciences, which was also called the College of Osteopathic Sciences, was established in 1967 by Peter Derig, a graduate of the Sydney College of Chiropractic, who disagreed with both the management and curriculum of his alma mater and wanted to create a school that stressed osteopathy, dietetics, and naturopathy (Committee of Inquiry, 1977:625). The Institute of Natural Health in the Glebe section of Sydney was originally created by Chris Dalton as the Alternative Health Centre and offered diplomas in natural therapeutics, osteopathy, and chiropractic (Committee of Inquiry, 1977:630). Mrs. P.H. Laws, a graduate of the Southern School of Naturopathy who disagreed with the philosophy and operation of her alma mater, established the Laws School of Naturopathy in her private clinic in Carnegie, Victoria (Committee of Inquiry, 1977:639). She offered a four year course in naturopathy and chiropractic. Other private natural therapy schools established during this period were the Queensland Institute of Natural Sciences (est. 1965), the New South Wales College of Naturopathic (est. 1967 and later called Health Schools Australia), the

College of Naturopathic Sciences (est. 1967) in Sydney, the Nature Care College of Naturopathic and Traditional Medicine (est. 1973) in New South Wales, and the Australian College of Natural Medicine (est. 1975) with campuses in Queensland and Victoria (Committee of Inquiry, 1977:625–642; Martyr, 2002:275).

Table 4 below presents a partial listing of naturopathic or natural therapy association that existed during the 1960s and 1970s. The Association of Natural Practitioners formed in 1970–1971 as an organization for graduates of the New South Wales College of Naturopathic Sciences (Committee of Inquiry, 1977:261). The Australian Council of Natural Therapies was created in December 1974 and merged with the South Pacific Federation of Natural Therapeutics to become the South Pacific Council for Natural Therapies in July 1975 (Jacka, 1998:39). This association sought to develop uniform educational standards among the fifteen naturopathic or natural therapy colleges in Australia and included the National Association of Naturopaths of Australia; the Australian Chiropractors, Osteopaths and Naturopathic Physicians Association; the South Australian Chiropractic Association; the Victorian Chiropractors Association; the Victorian Society of Specialist Osteopaths; the Southern School of Osteopathy; and the Canberra College of Natural Therapeutics; the Queensland Institute of Natural Science; the Windsor College of Osteopathy; the School of Herbal Medicine; and the New South Wales College of Naturopathic and Osteopathic Sciences (Committee of Inquiry, 1977:265). In its submission to the Federal Committee of Inquiry into Chiropractic, Osteopathy, and Naturopathy, the National Association of Naturopaths of Australia (1975:9) stated that there were at the time approximately 1000 practising chiropractors, osteopaths, and naturopaths which were represented by a dozen or so associations. The submission also states that most naturopaths were either osteopaths or chiropractors as well and that most chiropractors were naturopaths to a certain degree. Yet another umbrella organisation,

Table 4
Naturopathic or natural therapy associations

Association	Year established
National Herbalists' Association of Australia	1921
Australian Chiropractors, Osteopaths and Naturopathic Physicians Association	1936
Association of Natural Health Practitioners	1970–71
South Pacific Federation of Natural Therapeutics	early 1970s
Australian Naturopathic Physicians Association	1975
South Pacific Council for Natural Therapies	1975
Victorian Naturopathic Physicians and Chiropractors Association	1976

Source: Committee of Inquiry (1977:264–267)

the Australian Council for Natural Therapies consisted of various colleges, including the College of Naturopathy, Acupuncture Colleges (Australia), the Southern School of Naturopathy, and the NSW College of Osteopathy (National Association of Naturopaths of Australia, 1975:9).

Although herbalism has for long been an integral part of naturopathy as it has of Chinese medicine, some complementary practitioners emphasised Western herbal medicine. Herbalists organised themselves, in part to counteract the opposition of organised regular medicine or biomedicine and parts in part to seek statutory registration. The Australasian Union of Herbalists functioned for a short while in the early years of the twentieth century and was superseded by the Australian Herbalists Association (Bentley, 2005:45). The latter body campaigned against a bill introduced on behalf of pharmacists in 1925 by Stanley Argyle, a Nationalist Party parliamentarian in Victoria who went onto become premier in the 1930s. A combination of Labour opposition, fragmentation within the governing party, and a petition of some 6,000 signatures gathered by the Australian Herbalist Association contributed to the defeat of the bill which sought to restrict the practice of herbalists (Bentley, 2005:45). Even some upper-middle class intellectuals had signed the petition, a reflection of the fact that alternative practitioners often find support among certain 'strategic elites' (Freidson, 1970). According to Bentley,

> Under the combined assault of advances in orthodox medicine and the denigration from the medical profession the practice of herbalism slowly declined. Numbers in Melbourne remained in the 40s until the late 1940s, thereafter declining to a nadir of seven in the mid-1960s. The AHA also had a less than stellar career virtually disappearing from the public record after this and apparently amalgamating with the National Herbalists Association of Australia in the 1940s (Bentley, 2005:46).

The development of Chinese medicine in Australia

Traditional Chinese Medicine (TCM) was first introduced in Australia in the mid 1850s in the goldfields and other places where Chinese migrants settled in Australia (About AACMA, www.acupuncture.org.au, accessed 18/02/2009). Chinese medicine practitioners served patients in Victorian goldmining towns such as Ballarat and Bendigo and in Melbourne's Chinatown (Bentley, 2005:41). According to Bentley,

> Four Melbourne-based herbalists were listed in the first Sands and McDougall *Directory of Victoria* published in 1862. Over the succeeding years this figure grew steadily peaking at more than fifty in the

mid-1920s. These figures would only have represented a portion of practitioners as not all would have listed and there were many more in the country (Bentley, 2005:42).

Chinese medical practitioners served not only fellow Chinese but also European Australians. According to Phillips (1978:19), 'James Lam See had an enormous following in Bendigo, and drove the smartest buggy and pair in town. Wing Fat did equally well in Ballarat'.

Chinese herbalists introduced a treatment for diphtheria, a major disease in early Victoria. During the winter of 1873, Ah Sue, a Chinese herbalist based in Ararat, 'successfully treated 30 children suffering from diphtheria' (Tiqua, 2004:146). Lo Suai Sang, a Chinese medicine practitioner in the Ballarat gold fields, reportedly treated 65 cases of diphtheria within the span of three months sometime in the 1870s. Luo Kuai Sang practised Chinese medicine initially in South Ballarat and then in Melbourne suburb of Fitzroy (Tiqua, 2004:148). He specialised in internal medicine, treated many cases during the Victorian diphtheria epidemic, and also operated a herbal mail service (Tiqua, 2004:148–150). Luo along with Cheong Kee Chun were tried in May 1875 for allegedly using the title of 'Doctor' in violation of the Medical Practitioner Statute 1865. Whereas Luo was acquitted of wrong-doing, Cheong was fined. G. Tye Kee practiced Chinese medicine in Fitzroy from ca. 1897 to ca. 1952 and S.T. Goon practiced Chinese medicine in Melbourne proper from ca. 1927 to ca. 1972 (Bentley, 2005:42).

Summary

Biomedicine had indeed achieved clear-cut dominance over an array of alternative medical systems during the course of first half of the twentieth century. Certain alternative medical systems, such as homeopathy and electrotherapy, went into decline; others, such as naturopathy and Western herbalism, struggled but managed to survive, and yet others, such as chiropractic, osteopathy, and massage therapy, even grew and prospered. As subsequent chapters indicate, beginning in the 1960s various state governments and then in the 1970s, the Australian government began to conduct inquiries into various alternative medical systems, particularly chiropractic, osteopathy, homeopathy, and naturopathy. In part these inquiries were prompted by a growing popular interest in alternative medical systems within the context of the emergence of the holistic health movement.

Chapter 2

Chiropractic and osteopathy in Australia – recognition and funding

Introduction

In their drive for professionalisation and legitimacy, complementary or alternative health practitioners often emulate biomedicine by pursuing some form of licensure, certification, or registration from the state or recognition from an accrediting agency, even one internal to a specific complementary medicine group. Heterodox practitioners around the world have a long history of conducting intense campaigns to obtain statutory registration or licensure and have often found support among sympathetic politicians, many of whom have utilized alternative medicine to address their own ailments or those of family members. In the struggles between rival medical systems, the state, which holds the power to confer licensure, has tended historically to side with biomedicine. Statutory registration or licensure has played and continues to play a double-edged role in the development of complementary medical systems in the sense that it forces them to adopt aspects of biomedical theory and practice so that their students and practitioners can meet registration or licensing requirements. To avoid dramatic changes in the larger health care system, the legitimation granted to complementary medical systems extended by the state is generally only partial in that complementary practitioners are forced to comply with the structures, standards, and processes that are dominated by biomedicine. Cohen (2000:17) argues that while licensure or other forms of state credentialing purportedly serve to protect the public from charlatans and incompetent practitioners, it often fails to achieve this and essentially creates barriers to entry into a particular health occupation.

The Australian Constitution grants the power to create statutory practitioner registration to the state and territorial governments. Health occupations with statutory registration in every state and territory today include biomedicine, nursing, pharmacy, dentistry, physiotherapy, psychology, optometry, podiatry, and most recently chiropractic and osteopathy. In 2000 Victoria granted statutory registration for acupuncture and Chinese medicine. Khoury (2002), a herbalist, delineates three forms of regulations for health occupations in Australia, namely statutory registration, self-regulation, and co-regulation. He argues that eligibility for statutory registration tends to be premised on that belief that a particular health occupation or practice poses potential harm to patients.

Complementary practitioners may practice within certain limitations without statutory registration under the guidelines of Common Law. As in Britain, Australian Common Law is based upon judicial decisions or the application of the 'doctrine of precedent'. Complementary practitioners, however, are subject to 'criminal and civil law sanctions…, [including] being subject to action in negligence or for a criminal act' and 'consumer legislation such as the Fair Trading Act and Trade Practices Act' (Weir, 2000b:4–5).

Conversely, practitioners of more marginal medical systems, such as homoeopathy or various forms of bodywork, or groups of practitioners with limited training or education within a rising complementary medical system, such as naturopathy or acupuncture, may resist the social closure that statutory registration imposes. As Khoury observes,

> Advocates of self-regulation argue that CM is a relatively safe form of healthcare practice and therefore does not meet the criterion of statutory registation. They point out the restrictions and limitations on practice by an external authority with Minister-appointed delegates, high costs of membership and loss of control over the profession's direction and growth. Critics of self-regulation argue that it promotes anti-competitive behaviour, does not offer the consumer an adequate forum for dispute resolutions, lacks any legal underpinning, tends to be dominated by those with commericial interest, is too dependent on professional association politics, and has failed to advance the credit-ability of the profession (Khoury, 2002:43).

Both the Australian government and the various state governments have been reluctant to grant statutory registration to complementary practitio-ners along with certain conventional allied health professional groups and have tended to encourage them to engage in self-regulation. For example, the Victorian government encourages Aboriginal health workers, child-birth educators, 'Doula' birth helpers, hypnotherapists, massage therapists, naturopaths, optical dispensers, personal care attendants, ambulance offi-cers, counsellors, psychotherapists, herbalists, lactation consultants, music therapists, occupational therapists, and speech therapists to regulate their practice because 'non-compliance by members of [these groups with their] standards of practice are not catastrophic' (Carlton, 2003:126).

Co-regulation entails a mixture of self-regulation and statutory registra-tion in that criteria for practice are dictated by the health occupational group but with state support and recognition. Khoury (2002:43) maintains that '[c]o-regulation has successfully worked with CM [complementary medicine] products… where the Therapeutic Goods Administration and the industry association, the Complementary Health Council, have worked together to regulate supply, manufacture and advertising of therapeutic goods'.

As professionalised heterodox medical systems, chiropractic and osteopathy during the 1980s paved the way for the potential statutory recognition of other complementary medical systems. Thus far, however, only acupuncture and Chinese medicine in Victoria has been the only other complementary medical system to have obtained statutory registration in any state or territory. Nevertheless, as is demonstrated later in this book, various other complementary medicine professional groups, particularly those that collectively fall under the rubric of 'natural medicine' or 'natural therapies', have been lobbying various jurisdictions of the Australian state for statutory recognition. Bearing these more recent efforts in mind, it seems appropriate to begin the story of the drive for professionalisation and legitimacy on the part of complementary medical systems with the a narrative of how the chiropractic and osteopathic professions have achieved a relatively high degree of recognition within the context of the larger dominative medical system of Australia.

Parliamentary inquiries setting the stage for the statutory registration of chiropractic and osteopathy in Australia

The way for the eventual statutory registration of chiropractors and osteopaths was paved by a series of commissioned parliamentary investigations into the status of various alternative medical systems, particularly chiropractic, osteopathy, naturopathy, and homoeopathy. One of the first of these was the 'Royal Commission to Inquire into Matters Relating to Natural Therapists' in Western Australia (Guthrie, 1961). Sir Charles Henry Gairdner, the Lieutenant-General of Western Australia, appointed an investigative commission chaired by Hugh Norman Guthrie and several other members of the legislative assembly. The Commission considered four health care specialities, namely chiropractic, osteopathy, naturopathy, and dietetics. With respect to chiropractic, the Commission concluded that 'it would appear that harm, likely to be suffered by the patients from the activities of chiropractors, is comparatively slight' (Guthrie, 1961:11), and thereby recommended that the passage of legislation granting them statutory registration. Given the presence of only a few osteopaths in Western Australia, the Commission deferred on making a recommendation on passage of legislation that would have resulted in statutory registration for them. It also recommended statutory registration for dieticians on that proviso that a 'Dieticians' Board would register only dieticians having the qualification necessary to obtain appointment at major public hospitals', a condition that would bring dieticians under the direct supervision of biomedicine (Guthrie, 1961:16).

The Commission, however, expressed major misgivings about naturopathy. It argued that on the basis of the evidence presented 'that all the methods practised by naturopaths in Western Australia could not be said to be harmless' (Guthrie, 1961:12). It questioned the quality of naturopathic education not only in Australia but elsewhere in the world and criticised its modalities, particularly iridiagnosis, and concluded that 'naturopaths (to the extent that they exceed the ambit of chiropractic and dietetics,) should not be encouraged and, indeed, should be prohibited' (Guthrie, 1961:15). The Guthrie Report paved the way for Western Australia in 1964 becoming the first Australian jurisdiction to grant chiropractors statutory registration.

In 1973 the Victoria Parliament formed the Joint Select Committee on Osteopathy, Chiropractic, and Naturopathy that was chaired by H.R. Ward (1975). The Ward Committee also investigated the organizational, educational, and clinical aspects of Christian Science, herbalism, homoeopathy, and acupuncture in Victoria. It recommended the creation of Manipulative Therapy Board in Victoria with one division qualifying chiropractors and osteopaths and other physiotherapists and masseurs (Ward, 1975:vii). The Ward Committee also recommended that herbalists be registered in Victoria and that homeopathic practitioners 'should have completed a medical course in the allopathic field' (Ward, 1975:vii). With respect to naturopaths, the Committee rather vaguely recommended that '[a]ll persons who, in any way, purport to diagnose or prescribe treatments for physical or mental conditions should first be registered with the Department of Health' (Ward, 1975:vii). The Ward Committee recommended that chiropractors, osteopaths, and naturopaths, and physiotherapists undergo a 'common core of basic subjects in the first two years of tertiary education' (Ward, 1975:viii). Regarding acupuncture, it recommended that the Minister of Health appoint a committee to investigate both its clinical aspects and its training programs in Australia and abroad (Ward, 1975:vii). The recommendations of the Ward Committee were never implemented because they were superseded by those of the federal Committee of Inquiry into Chiropractic, Osteopathy, Homeopathy, and Naturopathy (1977). A committee of inquiry into chiropractic was also created in New South Wales in 1973 (Peters & Peters, 1985:170).

D.N. Everingham, the Minister of Health, formed the Committee in February 1974 at which time he invited Professor E.C. Webb, the Vice-Chancellor of Macquarie University in Sydney, to serve as its chair. Other members of the Committee were C.J. Cummins, former Director-General of Public Health of New South Wales; M.J. Rand, Professor of Pharmacology at the University of Melbourne; and R.H. Thorp, Professor Emeritus of

Pharmacology at the University of Sydney and Chairperson of the Council of Australian Consumers Association (Committee of Inquiry, 1977:1). The Committee interviewed numerous representatives from the various complementary medicine associations and schools and other experts and commissioned inspections of the various schools. The Committee produced a report of 930 pages detailing the historical, organizational, legal, and clinical aspects of chiropractic, osteopathy, homoeopathy, and naturopathy in Australia. Despite its strong biomedical bias, it constitutes an important baseline in the social historical study of complementary medicine in Australia.

The Committee proposed statutory registration of chiropractors and osteopathy and the creation of chiropractic and osteopathic training programs at a tertiary institution. In part because manipulative therapy became popular among physiotherapists, the Australian Physiotherapy Association opposed statutory recognition of chiropractors (O'Neill, 1994a:150). Indeed, Maitland, a leading physiotherapist-manipulator, called for the creation of manipulative therapy as a specialty of physiotherapy. Nevertheless, in 1978 Victoria and New South States became the first Australian jurisdictions to create statutory registration for chiropractors and osteopaths (Hawkins & O'Neill, 1990:36). Victoria formed the Chiropractors and Osteopaths Registration Board consisting of seven members, three of them heterodox practitioners, three biomedical physicians, and one a ministerial appointee (Willis, 1989a:189). This legislation essentially narrowed the scope of chiropractic care to musculoskeletal disorders along with some visceral and organic ones. Queensland passed the Chiropractors and Osteopaths Act in 1979, the Australian Capital Territory in 1983, and Tasmania in 1997 (Martyr, 2002:299). South Australia passed the Chiropractors Act in 1991 that also served to register osteopaths. Despite the fact that chiropractic and osteopathy achieved statutory registration in the face of biomedical opposition, this victory entailed considerable restriction of scope of practice (Clavarino & Yates, 1995:256).

In most state and territories, chiropractors and osteopaths may refer to themselves as 'Doctor' or 'Dr'. Western Australia and Queensland permit the use of the title Doctor if used with the qualifier chiropractor or chiropractic, or osteopath or osteopathy (Weir, 2000b:141–142). In May 1991 Parliament passed an amendment to the Health Insurance Act recognising the right of chiropractors to refer patients for x-rays (Willis, 1993).

The chiropractic scenario

In the mid-1970s, the chiropractic associations and schools depicted in Table 5 were in existence in Australia. The Webb Committee recommended statutory recognition for both chiropractic and osteopathy but emphasized

Table 5	Association	Year established
Australian Chiropractic Associations in the 1970s	Australian Chiropractors, Osteopaths, and Naturopathic Physicians Association	1936
	Australian Chiropractors' Association	1938
	Western Australian Chiropractors' Association	1957
	United Chiropractors' Association of Australasia	1961
	Southern Australian Chiropractic Association	1963
	Australian Association of Chiropractors	1965
	Victorian Society of Chiropractors	1974
	Victorian Chiropractors' Association	1975

Source: Committee of Inquiry (1977:261–267)

that only on the condition that such recognition should not 'imply that they were alternative health systems' (Committee of Inquiry, 1977: 128–129). It also recommended the creation of bachelor degrees for both. The Australian Federation of Chiropractors constituted an effort to unify the profession and eventually became the United Chiropractors Association of Australasia (Devereax, 1998:71). The Australian Chiropractors Association and New Zealand Association joined forces in 1975 in order to form the Australian Council on Chiropractic Education (Devereaux, 1998:75). The Chiropractic Society of Australia formed in November 1985 because various chiropractors felt that the mainstream of the ACA has been drifting away from straight chiropractic (O'Neill, 1994a:79). The new organization identified closely with the philosophy of the Sherman College of Straight Chiropractic in Spartanburg, South Carolina. After years of intense rivalry, in September 1990 the Australian Chiropractors' Association (est. 1938) and United Chiropractors Association of Australasia (est. 1961) merged into the Chiropractors' Association of Australia (www.chiropractors.asn.au, accessed 29/4/2004). It reports that it has some 1900 members.

Several chiropractic colleges, including the Sydney College of Chiropractic (est. 1933, the Chiropractic College of Australasia in Carnegie, Victoria, and the Chiropractic and Osteopathic College in Waysville, South Australia, were in existence during the mid-1970s (Committee of Inquiry, 1977:623–640). The International College of Chiropractic joined this list when the Australian Chiropractors'Association created it in 1975 (Committee of Inquiry, 1977:144). It taught students in association with Technicsearch, a commercial arm of the Royal Melbourne Institute of Technology, and shortly afterwards in partnership with the Preston Institute of Technology (Devereux, 1998:71; Kinney, 1975; Willis, 1989a:189). Two rival associations, namely the United Chiropractors Association of Australasia (UCAA) and the Australian Chiropractors' Association (ACA), pushed for statutory registration. The recommendation of the Webb committee that chiropractic education be situated in a public tertiary institution prompted a fierce struggle between the UCAA and ACA and various tertiary education institutions in Melbourne (O'Neill, 1995:440).

Whereas the UCAA wanted to see the development of more than one chiropractic program in a tertiary institution, the ACA favoured the creation of a single national chiropractic program at a tertiary institution and considered at one point the University of New England in Armidale, New South Wales, as being the site for such a program (O'Reilly, 1981:10–11). The UCA entered negotiations with the Cumberland College of Health Sciences and the University of New South Wales in the search for a new chiropractic program and also supported the candidacy of Lincoln Institute of Health Sciences, which already had a school of physiotherapy, as the site for a publicly supported a chiropractic training program. The Lincoln physiotherapists and the Australian Physiology Association vehemently opposed the proposed location of a chiropractic programme at the Lincoln Institute (O'Neill, 1995:153). Furthermore, the fact that Lincoln insisted that the word 'chiropractic' not appear on the name of the degree ruled this option out. The chiropractic profession contemplated the possibility of establishing a chiropractic programme at Griffith University in Queensland, but this proposal met with resounding opposition from the Queensland branch of the Australian Medical Association (O'Neill, 1995:160).

Eventually, the ACA came to support the candidacy of Preston Institute of Technology that already was teaching basic science courses for the ACA-affiliated International College of Chiropractic (O'Neill, 1995:440). The Tertiary Education Commission broke the deadlock between the rival associations by insisting upon a joint statement on the creation of a chiropractic program (O'Reilly, 1981:10). E.P. Devereaux, the UCAA President, and J.A. Sweaney, the ACA President, complied by advocating the creation of more than one chiropractic program at a public tertiary institution (Deveraux & Sweaney, 1981).

The new four-year undergraduate chiropractic program was situated at the Preston Institute of Technology in 1980, which was renamed the Phillips Institute of Technology in 1982 after it merged with a teachers' college (O'Neill, 1995:441). The ACA and the UCA formed the National Consultative Council in 1984, a move that eventually contributed to the establishment of one national chiropractic association in Australia (Portelli, 1985:16). Phillips eventually was absorbed by the Royal Melbourne Institute of Technology University in 1992.

The chiropractic school at the Preston Institute of Technology constituted the first instance world wide of a chiropractic program being embedded within a larger higher education institution. Even today, no US or Canadian chiropractic college has been successful in achieving affiliation with a public university, and only one other chiropractic college, namely the one at the Unification Movement-owned University of Bridgeport (Connecticut) in the United States, is affiliated with a larger university per se (Baer, 2001:82).

According to Campbell, Dillon and Polus (1982:26), the creation of ICC/PIT 'put the other Australian schools at a decided and academic disadvantage in terms of attracting students and government funding'. Of the thirteen Australian chiropractic colleges in existence in 1975, only the Sydney College of Chiropractic survived the creation of a chiropractic school at a tertiary institution. In 1982 the New South Wales Higher Education Board accredited the Graduate Diploma of Chiropractic from the Sydney College of Chiropractic (Devereaux, 1998:79). The Chiropractic College of Australasia in Melbourne and the Chiropractic and Osteopathic College in Adelaide closed their doors in 1978 and their students transferred to the International College of Chiropractic. The Sydney College of Chiropractic negotiated for its absorption into the University of New South Wales, the Institute of Technology (later University of Technology, Sydney), and Macquarie University with the latter eventually incorporating it in 1990 (Bolton, 1989:27)

The Royal Melbourne Institute of Technology has a five-year program in chiropractic. Macquarie University offers a three-year bachelors degree in chiropractic and an additional two-year masters degree in chiropractic. Murdoch University, a private institution in Perth, enrolled its first chiropractic schools in 2002 (Lawrence, 2002:28).

According to Hunter (2002:44), the incorporation of basic science courses has prompted the Australian chiropractic profession to place less emphasis on traditional chiropractic philosophy.

The Chiropractors' Association of Australia has a national board consisting of ten members (www.chiropractors.asn.au, accessed 20/7/2004, p. 1). It recognises that some members may have dual registration as chiropractors and osteopaths. Some 1950 of the approximately 2600 registered and domiciled chiropractors in Australia reportedly belong to CCA (Lawrence, 2002:30). The Council of Chiropractic Education Australasia (est. 2002) serves as the accrediting body of chiropractic schools in Australia and New Zealand (www.ccea.com.au accessed 6/11/2004).

The osteopathic scenario

Both the Australian Osteopathic Association and the United Osteopathic Physicians Guild supported the establishment of an osteopathic program at Phillips Institute of Technology (O'Neill, 1994a:46). The osteopathic profession, however, did not play a important role in the negotiations that led to the creation of a chiropractic program at Preston (Hawkins & O'Neill, 1990:39). The Preston Institute of Technology offered to create a separate osteopathy degree in collaboration with Australian Osteopathic Association (Hawkins & O'Neill, 1990:40). Chiropractors who supported the creation of an osteopathic program de-emphasized the differences between chiropractic and osteopathy. Despite the opposition of the ACA, the School of School of Chiropractic became the School of Chiropractic and Osteopathy at the Phillip Institute of Technology in 1986 (Hawkins & O'Neill, 1990:40). Aside from the United States where colleges of osteopathic medicine were created at six state universities between the late 1960s and mid-1970s and where osteopathy had evolved into osteopathic medicine and surgery or a parallel medical system to biomedicine with manipulative therapy essentially functioning as an adjunct rather than central modality, the osteopathic program at Phillip Institute of Technology constituted the first instance of a state-sponsored training program in osteopathy as a heterodox medical system per se in the world (Baer, 2001:59–61). The Royal Melbourne Institute of Technology, Victoria University, and the University of Western Sydney all operate five-year degree courses in osteopathy which lead to initially a bachelors degree and then to a masters degree (Kron, 2003:23).

The merger of chiropractic and osteopathic programs in the same school created some tensions in the sense that the osteopaths felt that they were being absorbed by the chiropractors (O'Neill, 1994a:188). Whereas the chiropractors tended to be enthusiastic about the inclusion of physiological therapeutics in the curriculum, the osteopaths were less enthusiastic about this development. Some chiropractors maintained that osteopaths 'latched onto the chiropractic achievement of course recognition without paying the costs that chiropractors had met in setting up the International College' (Hawkins & O'Neill, 1990:43). Conversely, many osteopaths fear absorption by chiropractic (Hawkins & O'Neill, 1990:41).

The Australian Osteopathic Association sponsors an evening seminar program three or four times per year in each state capital city by individual state branches (Education, p. 1, www.osteopathic.com.au/education_postgrad.htm, accessed 19/02/2009). It reportedly represents the majority of the some 650 osteopaths practicing in Australia (Kron, 2003:26). The AOA has its federal office in the Chatswood West section of Sydney and has branches in New South Wales, the Australian Capital Territory, Victoria, Tasmania, South Australia, Western Australia, the Northern Territory, and Queensland. The Sutherland Cranial Teaching Foundation of Australia and

New Zealand operates an annual basic course on cranio-sacral mechanism and is affiliated with the Sutherland Cranial Teaching Foundation. The Student Osteopathic Medicine Association of Australia has branches at the Royal Melbourne of Technology University, the University of Western Sydney, and Victoria University.

Osteopathic registration is covered under the following bodies: the Chiropractors & Osteopaths Board of the Australian Capital Territory; the Osteopaths Registration Board of New South Wales; the Chiropractors & Osteopaths Board of the Northern Territory; the Osteopaths Board of Queensland; the Chiropractors Board of South Australia; the Chiropractors and Osteopaths Registration Board of Tasmania; the Osteopaths Registration Board of Victoria; the Osteopaths Registration Board of Western Australia (Osteopaths Registration Board of Victoria, October 2003:5).

The AOA maintains close relationships with the General Osteopathic Council in the UK, the New Zealand Register of Osteopaths, and the American Academy of Osteopathy (the leading speciality body in osteopathic manipulation therapy in the United States), but not the American Osteopathic Association which has a policy of only recognizing graduates of the US osteopathic medical schools and biomedical physicians who have undergone training in manual medicine, such as at the London College of Osteopathic Medicine in London (Baer, 1984b).

Osteopathy is covered by various government-sponsored schemes, such as WorkCover and the Traffic Accident Commission (Lucas & Moran, 2003:273). Several private health insurance plans provide rebates for chiropractic and osteopathic services (Clavariono & Yates, 1995:261).

How similar or different are chiropractic and osteopathy from each other in Australia

Although for much of the twentieth century chiropractic and osteopathy overlapped with each other in Australia, most osteopaths seem to prefer to view themselves as a distinctive health occupation from chiropractors. Nevertheless, one place where the two groups still meet is within educational workshops and seminars operated by the Chiropractic & Osteopathic College of Australasia which evolved out of the Chiropractors and Osteopaths Musculo-Skeletal Interest Group (est. 1990) based at the Ringwood Clinic in Melbourne (About COCA, p. 1, www.coca.com/au, accessed 17/02/2009). COCA publishes the *Australasian Journal of Chiropractic and Osteopathy*. On the 'About' section of its website, the Australian Osteopathic Association seeks to address the question, 'What's the difference between osteopaths, chiropractors, and physiotherapists?' Its response to this query states,

It's not the role of any health professional to try to define what another health professional is, and what they do. If you want a definition, it would be best to ask people in those professions. What we can do is tell you about the defining characteristics of Osteopathy, which are its underlying philosophy and its broad range of techniques (www.osteopathic.com.au/about.htm, p. 2).

The AOA asserts that 'osteopaths can call upon what is probably the largest range of techniques used in any manual therapy', including massage and stretching techniques; articulation techniques, which entail mobilising joints through their range of motion; counterstrain techniques, which 'achieve release of restriction by placing the affected joint or muscle in a position of comfort, while applying a 'counter' stretch to the antagonists of the tight muscles;' functional techniques 'involving gentle mobilisation of joint in order to release restrictions in movement; manipulation; cranial manipulation; and stretching of visceral areas' (www.osteopathic.com.au/about.htm, pp. 3–5, accessed 17/02/2009).

Summary

The Australian Government and various state governments have, since the 1960s, recognised the wide spread utilisation of complementary medicine among Australians and have grappled with this phenomenon, including to which complementary systems statutory registration should be granted, whether to fund complementary training programs in public tertiary institutions, and finally to include certain complementary therapies as eligible for Medicare rebates. With respect to all of these points, chiropractic and osteopathy constitute success stories in that they enjoy statutory registration in all political jurisdictions, have their training programs embedded only in public universities, and a few years ago qualified for partial Medicare rebate payments – however, only with the approval of a general practitioner. Furthermore, both chiropractic and osteopathy find themselves situated between heterodoxy and orthodoxy and have taken on many aspects of biomedicine both physically and therapeutically. Indeed, there appears to even be some debate as to whether they constitute complementary medical systems per se.

Chapter 3

Naturopathy, acupuncture, Chinese medicine and other holistic health practices

Introduction

The holistic health movement began to emerge on the US West Coast, especially the San Francisco Bay Area, in the early 1970s, but quickly spread to other parts of the United States and also other countries, especially Anglophone ones (namely Canada, Britain, Australia, and New Zealand), but also Western European countries, such as Germany, the Netherlands, and Denmark. It began as a popular movement that in various ways challenged the bureaucratic, high-tech and iatrogenic aspects of biomedicine. It drew upon the hippie or counter-cultural movement, the human potential movement, Eastern metaphysics, the environmental movement, and the feminist movement. The holistic health movement was by no means a monolithic phenomenon and varied considerably from society to society. It encompassed numerous alternative medical systems, such as homeopathy, herbalism, naturopathy, and bodywork, with divergent philosophical perspectives. Although it appeared to have its strongest expression in Western societies, it also drew heavily from various Eastern healing systems, such as Chinese medicine and Ayurveda. To a large extent, the holistic health movement overlapped with the New Age movement that also became very popular in particularly Western societies. Like the holistic health movement, New Ageism focuses upon a balance in the interaction of mind, body, and spirit in its attempts to achieve experiential health and well-being. New Ageism also incorporates many therapeutic techniques and practices, including meditation, guided visualization, channelling, psychic healing, and neo-shamanism.

Scott (1999) asserts that proponents of 'holistic health' or 'holistic medicine' appear to be operating with three different conceptions of it. All of these assert that they focus on the whole person in that each asserts to a greater or lesser degree: that it takes 'some (or all) of the body, mind, emotions, spirit, environment, and social context into account (Scott, 1999:136); and that it shifts the locus of control in the healer–patient relationship towards patient, with the latter serving as a facilitator or teacher.

The first conception focuses on the ill or disabled body as an expressive vehicle which uses pain and other forms of disability to communicate psychosocial conflict (Scott, 1999:136–138). The second conception is an ecological or public health model that stresses preventive health and concerns social and environmental factors in disease etiology and hearkens back to nineteenth-century social medicine (Scott, 1999:138–139). The third approach stresses spiritual, transpersonal or sacred concerns as an essential component of achieving wholeness or even 'holiness' (Scott, 1999:139–141). Needless to say, there is a certain degree of overlap among all three approaches.

The holistic health movement overlaps considerably with the New Age movement that appears to have emerged in the late 1960s and early 1970s, particularly in North America and Great Britain, but also other parts of the world (Prince & Riches, 2000). York (1995:42) characterizes the New Age movement as 'especially an American-Canadian-British-Dutch-West German-Australian-New Zealand phenomenon'. Despite a strong niche in particular in Anglo phone countries, the New Age movement seeks to bridge East–West connections. According to Melton, Clark, and Kelly (1991:169), the 'New Age and Holistic Health movements in theory exist independently, but are united philosophically by one central concept: the individual person is responsible for his or her own life and for seeking out the means of transformation needed to achieve a better quality of life'. New Agers seek to create a 'new planetary culture', characterized by inner-peace, wellness, unity, self-actualization, and attainment of higher consciousness. They believe that most, if not all, religions contain a hidden core of authentic spirituality.

Healing, including the notion of holistic health, pervades the New Age movement. New Age healing includes a seemingly endless proliferation of therapeutic techniques and practices, such as centering, channelling, astral projection, guided visualization, iridiology, reflexology, chromotherapy, rebirthing, and healing with the power of pyramids and crystals. New Agers tend to see matter and energy as intricately intertwined and believe that the latter is a vital component in efforts to achieve self-actualization and transcendence over the mundane nature of everyday life. Levin and Coreil (1986) delineate three types of New Age healing approaches: (1) body-centered groups that stress secular and Western therapies, such as Silva mind control, that seek psychosomatic health; (2) mind-oriented groups that draw on Western metaphysical or religious therapies, such as those associated with Theosophy and Anthroposophy; and (3) soul-oriented groups that stress Buddhist and Hindu mystical practices, such as meditation.

While the route of diffusion of the holistic health/New Age movement from North America to Australia has yet to be delineated in detail, Martyr observes that,

> The social revolution of the 1960s in the United States generated a variety of related interconnected movements in Australia, including rural resettlement, communal living, permaculture, natural healing, environmentalism, the new age, nuclear disarmnament, alternative religions, alternative schooling, personal development, and arts and crafts. Some of these revived older ideas – among the alternative religions were spiritualism, the teachings of Swedenborg and theosophy; among the natural healing therapies were herbalism and homeopathy (Martyr, 2002:268).

Other complementary medical systems that struck a popular chord during this time period included naturopathy, Chinese medicine, various forms of bodywork, and midwifery.

The rejuvenation of naturopathy and the natural therapies in Australia

While the terms 'naturopath' and 'naturopathy' continue to be used in a variety of contexts, including academic programs and professional associations, the terms 'natural therapies' or 'natural medicine' have become commonplace and are applied to a wide array of therapeutic systems, including Western herbalism, acupuncture, massage therapy, homeopathy, reflexology, and aromatherapy (Wiesner, 1981). During the late 1960s and early 1970s, the 'new style flower children' began to join the 'old style straight-backed nature cure adherents' as practitioners of natural medicine (Evans, 2000b:236).

The natural therapies or natural medicine were represented by numerous associations, including the Australian Traditional-Medicine Society, the Australian Natural Therapies Association, the Alumni Association of Natural Medicine Practitioners, the Australasian Federation of Natural Therapists, and the Australian Council of Natural Therapies. The Australian Naturopathic Practitioners Association (www.anpa.asn/anpa) was established in 1975 and claims to be the longest standing association of naturopathy in Australia. This association resulted as a merger of the National Association of Naturopaths (NAN) and the Australian Naturopathic Physicians Association Limited. NAN had earlier been known as the National Association of Naturopaths, Osteopaths, and Chiropractors and ANPAL as the Australian Chiropractors, Osteopaths and Naturopathic Association Limited (Jacka, 2005:9). According to Jacka,

> During the 1980s, ANTA broadened its membership to include other modalities such as acupuncture and massage. It was successful

in being the first association to gain partial rebates on consultations for its naturopathic members from a number of health funds. Rebates for acupuncturist and massage patients followed. ANTA also began comprehensive accreditation processes for colleges (Jacka, 2005:10).

The Australian naturopathic network (www.ann.com.au) was established in 1998.

Numerous new private naturopathic or natural therapy colleges were established during the 1970s and 1980s. These included the Nature Care College of Naturopathic and Traditional Medicine (est. 1973) in New South Wales, the Australian College of Natural Medicine (est. 1975) in Queensland and Victoria, the International Academy of Nutrition (est. 1980) in New South Wales, the Australasian College of Natural Therapies (est. 1981) in New South Wales, the ACT College of Natural Therapies (est. 1985), and the NSW School of Natural Medicine (est. 1987) (Martyr, 2002:272–276).

A considerable amount of overlap developed between naturopathy and Western herbalism beginning in the late 1960s. According to Hunter (1991:278), 'Western herbalism in Australia has in one sense diminished, in that it is now more likely to be incorporated into a broader natural therapies practice'. The National Herbalists Association of Australia (www.nhaa. org.au) includes many naturopaths within its ranks and has several 'state' chapters, namely NSW Central Coast, NSW Northern Rivers, NSW State, West Australia, Queensland Sunshine Coast, South Australia, and Western Victoria. It has developed standards covering training and therapeutic philosophy and conducted a major review of Education and Course Accreditation during 2002 and accredits courses but not training institutions. Its members are recognised by the Australian Taxation Office for exemption from the General Sales Tax. A postal survey of the NHAA membership, in which 58 percent of the members responded, revealed that Western herbal practitioners in Australia tend to utilise individualised herbal formulae, often administered in the form of liquid herbal extracts, rather than single herbs (Casey, Adams, & Sibbritt, 2007).

The Australian Complementary Health Association constitutes a forum where natural therapists and consumers converge, largely through in the form of a journal titled *Diversity: Natural & Complementary Health* (www. diversity.org.au, accessed 3/01/2009). ACHA is the creation of Jocelyn Bennett, a journalist and promoter of complementary medicine. The association views itself as a body of 'health consumers and practitioners who encourage a diversity of approaches to healing and promote the integration of complementary therapies into the mainstream health system' (About diversity, www.diversity.org.au, page 4). The journal's editorial board includes a listing of 'who's who's' in the world of Australian complementary medicine, including Alan Bensoussan (Head of Chinese Medicine at the University of Western Sydney), Sue Evans (a lecturer in herbal medicine at Southern Cross University), Ian Gawler (the Director of the Gawler Foundation in Yarra Junction, Victoria), Judy Jacka (Ringwood Natural Therapies), Paul Orrock (a senior lecturer in naturopathy and osteopathy at Southern Cross University), and Charlie Xue, the Head of the Chinese Medicine Unit at the Royal Melbourne Institute of Technology).

The expansion of Chinese medicine and acupuncture in Australia

Despite its prior presence, Chinese medicine and acupuncture attained popularity under the umbrella of the holistic health movement and in wake of US President Nixon's visit to China, resulting in widespread exposure of the use of acupuncture as an effective form of anesthesia. Chinese medicine also grew in popularity during the 1970s and 1980s due to the influx of Chinese medicine practitioners from China and Vietnam and readier access to raw Chinese herbs. One source maintains that Eddie Wong of the Taiwan Institute of Chinese Medicine brought acupuncture to Australia in 1970 (Acupuncture Association of Australia 2000:7).

The Chinese medicine and acupuncture profession has been and continues to be fractionated among its various schools and associations. O'Neill (1994a:107) asserts that 'traditional acupuncturists were even in greater organisational disarray' than chiropractors. Russell Jewell, a chiropractor, created Acupuncture Colleges (Australia) in Sydney in 1969 (O'Neill, 1994a:vi). The Acupuncture Association of Australia reportedly was formed in 1972 at a meeting at the Sydney College of Chiropractic by 31 chiropractors and osteopaths who had graduated from Acupuncture Colleges of Australia (Acupuncture Association of Australia, 2000:9). Peter Denig, a naturopath, osteopath, and acupuncturist, served as its first president.

The Australian Acupuncture College in Melbourne emerged as a separate institution but maintained a close relationship with the Sydney school (O'Neill, 1994a). An acupuncture college was also established in Brisbane during the early 1970s (About AACMA, www.acupuncture.org.au, accessed 18/02/2009). The NSW College of Natural Therapies reportedly created the 'first fulltime, four year course for an Australian Diploma in Traditional Chinese Medicine' in 1980 (Wiesner, 1989:57).

Table 6 depicts a selected listing of acupuncture and Chinese medicine Associations in Australia.

Table 6	Associations
Selected listing of acupuncture and TCM associations*	Acupuncture Association of Australia, New Zealand, and Asia
	Acupuncture Association of South Australia
	Acupuncture Association of Victoria
	Acupuncture Ethics and Standards Organisation
	Alliance of Chinese Medicine Associations Australia
	Aust-China Acupuncture and Chinese Medicine Association
	Australian Acupuncture Association
	Australian Acupuncture Federation
	Australian College of Acupuncturists
	Australian Council for Traditional Chinese Medicine Education
	Australian Medicine and Acupuncture Society of Australia
	International Acupuncture Association
	NSW Association of Chinese Medicine
	Traditional Medicine of China Society Australia

*Source: Australian Acupuncture and Chinese Medicine Association (2001:viii)

The Australian Acupuncture Association was formed in 1973 (About AACMA, www.acupuncture.org.au). The Webb Committee (Committee of Inquiry, 1977:37) observed that that its members were 'locally trained fringe practitioners who are eclectic in their choice of names and disciplines, sometimes advertising their services as chiropractors, osteopaths, or acupuncturists' (Committee of Inquiry, 1977:37). Many of these practitioners had obtained training from F.G. Roberts, the Chiropractic College of Australasia, or the Southern School of Naturopathy (Committee of Inquiry, 1977:37). In January 1977, the Acupuncture Specialists Practitioners Association reportedly had 98 members, primarily in New South Wales.

Acupuncture Colleges formed the Acupuncture Ethics and Standards Organisation (AESO) in 1977 as a mechanism for certifying practitioners so that their patients could obtain reimbursement from private health insurance plans (Wiesner, 1989:57). The colleges and the AESO created that Australian Council of Acupuncture and Traditional Chinese Medical Education (O'Neill, 1994a:113). On 1 March 1995 the Australian Acupuncture Association and the AESO merged and in 1996 the new Australian Acupuncture and Chinese Medicine Association (AACMA) absorbed the Acupuncture Association of South Australia (About AACMA). In 1998 the AAA changed its name to Australian and Chinese Medicine Association that claims to represent over 90 percent of 'qualified' acupuncture and Chinese medicine practitioners in Australia, of which there are reportedly 1700–1800 (About AACMA, pp. 2–3). The AACMA 'recognises graduates of four to five year Australian bachelor degree programs in acupuncture and/or Chinese herbal medicine and some sub-degree programs that are currently applying for bachelor degree level and/or for articulation with a recognised bachelor degree program (Studying TCM, p. 1, www.acupuncture.org.au, accessed 18/02/2009). The Australian Chinese Medicine Education & Research Council (est. 1995) consists of: academics, researchers, and practitioners; an advisory body on TCM education, research and practice; connections with the profession, government, and related health bodies; and members on executive body, board and committees (Australian Acupuncture and Chinese Medicine Association, www.acupuncture.org.au, accessed 18/8/2004. There reportedly were 23 Chinese medicine and acupuncture associations in the mid-1990s (Bensoussan & Myers, 1996:135).

The Acupuncture College (est. 1969) was the first acupuncture college established in Australia (Wiesner, 1989:57). The Federation of Acupuncture Teaching Institutions was established by eight major teaching colleges in Australia in 1980 (Wiesner, 1989:57). The Australian Acupuncture College in Sydney became part of University of Technology, Sydney which offers the Bachelor of Applied Science (Acupuncture). Victoria University of Technology absorbed in 1992 its sister college in Melbourne and offers the Bachelor Degree in Health Science (Acupuncture). The Royal Melbourne Institute of Technology developed a master's degree in acupuncture. Thirteen Australian universities and private colleges offered teaching programs in TCM during the mid-1990s (Bensoussan & Myers, 1996:157).

The Ward Committee reported that physiotherapists, biomedical physicians, and chiropractors were all utilising acupuncture by the 1960s (Ward, 1975:37). A group consisting primarily of chiropractors created the Acupuncture Association of Australia in 1972 (Wiesner, 1989:57). Biomedical physicians specializing in acupuncture established the Australian Medical Acupuncture Society in 1973 (Wiesner, 1989:57). The Australian Natural Therapists Association formed an acupuncture branch in 1975 (Wiesner, 1989:83).

The development of other complementary medical systems

In addition to chiropractic, osteopathy, Chinese medicine and acupuncture, and naturopathy, numerous other complementary medical systems exist in Australia. These include homeopathy, various forms of body work, and a wide array of religious healing systems and folk medical systems.

Homeopathy

Despite the fact that homeopathy has by and large become 'subsumed under the umbrella of natural therapies' in Australia, there are a number of distinct homeopathic bodies in the country (Clavarino & Yates, 1995:257). The oldest of these is the Australian Institute of Homeopathy, which was established in 1946 (Martyr, 2002:279). Other homeopathic organizations include the Australian Homeopathic Association, the Australian Council for Homeopathy (Victoria), the Australian Homeopathic Association (New South Wales), the Australian Homeopathic Association (South Australia), and Australian Association of Professional Homeopaths (Martyr, 2002:279). The Australian Homeopathic Association formed in 1995 from a merger of the New South Wales, South Australia and Victoria/Tasmania branches of the Australian Federation of Homeopaths, the Australian Society of Homeopaths (Queensland), and the Oceanic Homeopathic Research Foundation (Western Australia) and further mergers in 1997 with Australian Federation of Homeopaths in Queensland and Western Australia and with Homoeopathic Association of New South Wales (www.homeopathy.oz.org/intro.html, accessed 18/02/2009). The Australian Register of Homoeopaths was created in 1999 as a voluntary registry and an accrediting body for various homoeopathic training programs or schools (www.aroh.com.au, accessed 5/11/2004). Its board consist of representatives from various homoeopathic associations.

Homoeopathic education has in large part been incorporated into the curricula of the broader natural therapies schools, such as the Adelaide Training College of Complementary Medicine, the Australian College of Natural Therapies, and the Australasian College of Natural Therapies. Notable exceptions include the Victorian College of Classical Homeopathy (est. 1989), the Australasian College of Hahnemannian Homoeopathy (est. 1990), the Oceanic Institute of Classical Homoeopathy in Victoria Park, Western Australia, the Sydney College of Homoeopathic Medicine, and the Academy of Homoeopathic Medicine in Highgate Hill, Queensland (Martyr, 2002:279–80). Many homeopaths are interested in Bach flower remedies. Ian White, a herbalist and naturopath, has elaborated upon Bach flower remedies by developing a therapeutic modality called Australian bush flower essences (www.ausflowers.com.au, accessed 10/11/2008). He argues that Australian plants contain the potential to improve sexuality, communication, self-esteem, creativity, spirituality, and emotional well-being.

Bodywork

Massage therapy underwent a revival during 1970s within the context of the holistic health movement (Bentley, 2000:18). Today, the massage profession is self-regulating in Australia and requires certification involving a one year of study (Tuchtan, 2003:241). Massage associations include the West

Australian Association of Masseurs (est. 1968), the Association of Remedial Masseurs (est. 1972), and the Massage Association of Australia (est. 1990). The website of the MAA indicates that in 2001 there were 131 Australian institutions offering programs of study in massage therapy courses (Martyr, 2002:300). Schools of massage therapy include the Malvern School of Massage and Kinesiology (est. 1984) in Victoria; the Australian College of Tactile Therapies (est. 1984) in South Australia; the School of Integrated Body Therapy (est. 1985) in New South Wales; the School of Therapeutic Massage; the Gwinganna Academy of Remedial Therapies (est. 1988) in New South Wales; the Taree School of Holistic Massage (est. 1989) in New South Wales (Martyr, 2002:301).

Numerous other types of bodywork associations and schools exist in Australia. The Shiatsu Therapy Association of Australia (est. 1986) has accredited the following institutions for teaching shiatsu: Nature Cure College in Sydney; the Zen Renaissance Centre at Bondi Junction (Sydney); Australian Shiatsu College in Collingwood, Victoria; Shiatsu Australia in Caulfield South, Victoria (est. 1978); and the Queensland College of Oriental Medicine – Sunshine Coast Campus in Buderim (www.staa.org. au, accessed 10/11/2004). The Tai Chi Association of Australia (est. 1999) grew out of a workshop run by Paul Lam in Sydney (www.taichiaustralia. com, accessed 10/11/2008).

George Goodheart, a chiropractor from Detroit in the US, developed kinesiology during the 1930s as a form of bodywork that drew insights from Eastern mind–body medicine. The Australian Kinesiology Association (www.aka-oz.org). Kinesiology Schools Australia has branches in Melbourne, Sydney, Perth, Brisbane, and Byron Bay (www.kinesiology. com.au). Kinesiology Connection in Melbourne is a centre and college affiliated with the Kinesiology Schools Australia.

Tom Bowen, a self-educated osteopath, created a distinctive form of bodywork that entails working with energy fields. The Bowen Therapists Foundation of Australia (www.bowen.asn.au) represents Bowen therapists. The Bowen School of Western Australia and International School of Bowen Therapy in Armadale, Victoria offer training in Bowen Therapy.

Yoga has become highly popular in Australia as it has around much of the world. The Australian Institute of Yoga Therapy offers the Advanced Diploma of Yoga Teaching that is accredited by Victorian Qualifications Authority and the Australian National Training Authority (www.australian-institute-yoga.com.au). The course is offered in Sydney, Melbourne, and Southeast Queensland. The Pilates Institute of Australasia is based in Sydney. Allan Menezes developed Pilates Method in Australia and other bodywork techniques (www.pilates.net, accessed 10/11/2008). The Institute offers courses in Melbourne, Brisbane, Perth, and Cairns as well as Auckland in New Zealand.

Reflexology originated as zone therapy, a therapeutic system that was developed by William Fitzgerald in the United States. Eunice Ingham, a student of Fitzgerald, elaborated upon zone therapy by developing an anatomical map of the foot being overlaid onto the foot. Reflexology is taught in both private natural therapy colleges, such as the Nature Care College of Naturopathic and Traditional Medicine in Sydney, and specific reflexology schools, such as the Australian School of Reflexology in Nords Wharf, NSW. Moss Arnold developed a unique form of reflexology, called chi-reflexology, that incorporates aspects of Traditional Chinese Medicine. He founded the Australian College of Chi-Reflexology in 1995 (www.chi-reflexology. com.au, accessed 27/10/2004). The Reflexology Association of Australia (est. 1989/1990) serves as the primary organization for reflexologists in Australia (www.reflexology.org.au) and reportedly has about 900 members (Reflexology World Magazine, www.reflexologyworld.com/australi1.htm, accessed 19/11/2008). It consists of several state associations which have their own constitutions. It publishes a quarterly magazine titled *Footprints*. The Australian Traditional Medicine Society lists some 300 reflexologists among its members. The Professional Reflexology Association has about twenty members, most of whom are nurses. Reflexologists obtain their training in a diversity of programs, ranging from weekend workshops up to 200 hours of training in complementary medicine schools of one sort or other.

Religious healing systems

Spiritualism and spiritual healing have been practised in Australia since 1860s (Martyr, 2002:305). William Henry Terry, a Unitarian, abandoned his drapery business in order to operate a Spiritualist bookshop and healing practice on Russell Street in Melbourne (Sparrow & Sparrow, 2001:204). He reportedly supported women's liberation, vegetarianism, and temperance and opposed anti-Chinese discrimination (Sparrow & Sparrow, 2001:205). The Victorian Association of Progressive Spiritualists grew out of a meeting at Trades Hall in Melbourne in 1870 and claimed to have some 300 members and meetings of more than 1000. Spiritualists created a string of lyceums in Melbourne, Richmond, Bendigo, Stallwell, and Castlemaine (Sparrow & Sparrow, 2001:206–207). Christian Science diffused to Australia from the United States and reportedly 'by 1910, there were 29 accredited practitioner/healers, of whom two-thirds were women' (Sherwood, 2005:133).

Locke (1993) conducted an ethnographic study of the Sanctuary, a Spiritualist congregation established by Trudy Lucas, an English immigrant, in Freemantle, the port city of Perth, in 1954 and moved to Mosman in 1957. The healing rituals of the group entailed transmitting spiritual power from the Masters, including the Great Power and Jesus Christ, were conducted on Wednesdays in two services, one from 2 to 5 pm and the other from 7 to 10 pm. The mediums in the congregation also provided counselling for a wide range of problems, particularly marital, sexual, and financial ones. Trudy assumed an isolationist stance toward other Spiritualist congregations in the area but managed to attract a fair number of followers, with some 120 people generally attending her services. Following the death of her husband in 1964, she delegated more authority to other mediums which consisted exclusively of ageing women.

While most mainstream congregations in Australia tend to de-emphasize religious healing, one exception is Christ Church Saint Lawrence in Sydney established by Anglican priest John Hope who reportedly still conducts healing services (Martyr, 2002:307). Conversely, Pentecostalism, an international religious healing sect, constitutes one of the fast growing religious movements in Australia (Black, 1991:106). The Australian Census reported an increase from 38,393 Pentecostal church members in 1976 to 107,007 Pentecostal church members in 1986. A.C. Valdez, an American, served a pivotal role in the creation of the Assemblies of God in Australia (Hughes, 1996:46). Fredrick Van Dyke, a South African, established Pentecostal congregations and association that eventually became part of the Australian branch of the US-based Church of the Foursquare Gospel. British Pentecostals were involved in the formation of the Apostolic Church and New Zealander Phil Pringle established the Christian City Churches International. Other Pentecostal bodies formed by immigrants include the Finnish Pentecostal Churches of Australia, the Slavic Evangelical Pentecostal Church of Australia, the Hope Church of God (Thai-based), and the True Jesus Church (Chinese-based) (Hughes, 1996:46–47).

Yet another religious healing system is Scientology that was introduced as Dianetics to Australia in the early 1950s, first in Melbourne and later in Sydney (Kohn, 1991:135). It was officially recognised in a High Court decision in 1983 as Church of the New Faith and has reportedly seen thousands take its courses.

As part of the larger human potential movement, *Est* or Erhard Seminars Training, yet another American import, began offering courses in Sydney in 1982 (Kohn, 1991:135). It was renamed Forum in 1985 in Australia and claimed to have inducted about 9000 or 10,000 Australians into its courses.

Like North America and Europe, New Age religious groups constitute on of the fastest growing categories of religious groups in Australia

(Bouma, 2006:92–93, 165–166). The New Age movement has overlapped to a large extent with the holistic health movement. At any rate, New Age healing incorporates various therapeutic techniques and practices, including centering, channelling, astral projection, chromotherapy, rebirthing, and healing with the power of pyramids and crystals. It often incorporates techniques from earlier therapeutic systems, such as Ayurveda, yoga, shiatsu, reflexology, polarity therapy, iridology, shamanism, and other Indigeneous healing systems. [See also 'Healing with crystals' by Linda Johnson, 5 Aug 2004 (New Age of Ascension, www.newage.com.au).]

While apparently the *didjeridu* did not appear to have had a therapeutic significance for Aboriginal peoples in the past, New Ageism has incorporated it in its 'psychotechnologies of healing' (Neuenfeldt, 1998). Important sources of New Age discourse on the *didjeridu* include magazines, such as *The Wings of Eagles*, the cover notes for recordings, promotional materials, songs and albums, and New Age books such as Marlo Morgan's *Mutant Message from Down Under*. The Mind, Body and Spirit Festival which is held in Australian capital cities annually is an important venue for the New Age movement. According to Kohn,

> Around 200 exhibitors gather to ply their wares… In addition to these stalls, there are scores of guest gurus, local and international, who are on hand to give workshops, lectures and mini-courses on topics as wide ranging as ecognising angels in one's life, gaining a working knowledge of the powers of the Four Directions, channelling, mediumship and psychic development, ceremonial circles, colour waves of being, environmental spirituality, gems and crystals, and tantric sex (Kohn, 1996:158).

International New Ager speakers visiting Australia regularly include Deepak Chopra, Michael Rowland, Denise Lim, and Jean Huston. In his social profile of New Agers in Melbourne, Possamai (2000:373) found that 31 percent of his informants mentioned 'alienation as an everyday life crisis' for them. He also found that most of his interviewees tend to move from one group to another.

Folk medical systems

Given that Australia has evolved particularly since World War II into a multiethnic society, undoubtedly numerous folk medical systems exist there. Of these, Aboriginal folk medicine has received the greatest attention, particularly on the part of social anthropologists (Berndt, 1964). John Cawte (1974) reported that some three decades ago 'not a few Aboriginal doctors remain in remote Australia'. He interviewed eight Walbiri healers at Yuendumu about their illness beliefs and curing techniques (Cawte, 1974:41). Somewhat later, Janice Reid (1983) conducted research on the Indigenous medical system of the Yolngu people in Northeast Arhnem Land situated in the Northern Territory. She reports that the Aboriginal doctor and Indigenous concepts of sickness and curing are still an integral part of life in many Aboriginal communities. Indeed, the North Territory's Department of Health has employed Aboriginal healers and developed a program to collect and identify Indigenous herbal medicinal plants. Reid located and interviewed four Aboriginal Yolgnu healers or *marrnggitj* in the Yirrkala environs, two of them men, one of them a young boy, and one of them a woman. Finally, as a multi-ethnic society, Australia has numerous folk medical systems.

As noted earlier, the Chinese brought their traditional medical system to Australia beginning in the late nineteenth century when they immigrated in order to work in the gold fields of Victoria. Manderson and Matthews (1981, 1985) report that traditional medical beliefs and practices persist among Vietnamese immigrants because they provide cultural continuity in difficult situations. Big Leung (2008) also has examined Chinese folk medicine in a similar light among Chinese immigrants from various countries. With respect to another Asian immigrant group, Han (2000) observes that the Korean community in Australia did not even have either an herbal doctor or acupuncturist until 1980. Undocumented Korean migrants, however, sought herbal medicine and acupuncture in China Town when in acute pain.

Unfortunately virtually no scholarly research has been conducted on either Anglo-Australian folk medicine or the folk medical systems of the many ethnic groups, such as the Italians, the Greeks [See Bottley (1976) on health beliefs among immigrant Greeks], the Macedonians, the Lebanese, the Indians, and the Sudanese, found in Australia. This is quite in contrast to the United States where numerous studies have been conducted on various folk medical systems, such as Southern Applachian herbal medicine, African American folk medicine, *curanderismo* among Mexican Americans, *espiritismo* among Puerto Ricans, *santeria* among Cuban Americans, Chinese folk medicine, and Hmong folk medicine (Baer, 2001). In large part, a major reason for this is the fact that the United States as a country of some 300 million people has many more scholars investigating folk medicine than does Australia as a country of some 21 million people.

Studies of complementary medicine utilization in Australia

Numerous studies examining patient utilization of complementary medicine in Australia have been conducted since the early 1980s. The Australian

Bureau of Statistics (1983) conducted a survey in which extrapolated that 27,800 (0.8 percent) of Victorians had consulted a naturopath, herbalist, or acupuncturist in the two weeks prior to a 1983 interview. This percentage increased to 2.5 percent when chiropractors and osteopaths were included under the rubric of complementary practitioners. The study also indicated that twice as many females as males consulted naturopaths, herbalists, and acupuncturists. The Social Development Committee (1986), headed up by J.L. Dixon, conducted a study based upon both a telephone survey and interviews that indicated that during the previous five years,

> 22 percent of Victorians have used an alternative medicine practitio-
> ner (naturopath, homeopath, herbalist, iridologist and acupunctur-
> ist), or an osteopath or chiropractor who uses alternative medicine
> practices. Females, especially those in the workforce, are more likely
> to have used an alternative medicine practitioner. On the other hand,
> people in the 18–24 age group, those presently out of work force and
> people from lower blue collar households were relatively less likely to
> have used an alternative medicine practitioner (Social Development
> Committee, 1986:30).

Lloyd, Lupton, Wiesner, and Hasleton (1993:135) conducted a cross-sectional survey of 289 patients from eight Sydney practices providing a range of complementary modalities. They obtained the names and addresses of practitioners affiliated with the Australian Natural Therapists Association, the National Herbalists Association of Australia, and the Australian Traditional-Medicine Society. The therapists who agreed to participate in the survey or their receptionists provided a copy of a questionnaire to all patients as they arrived over period of three weeks. Ninety four percent of the 306 patients approached completed the questionnaire. Lloyd et al. (1993) found that majority of patients came from a narrow range of socio-economic backgrounds. Forty-five percent of the sample had attained some level of tertiary education. Seventy-one of the respondents were women which reflected the overall Australian pattern of health service utilisation on basis of gender (Lloyd, 1993:138). Forty-five percent were living alone, a level well above national figure of 14 percent obtained in the 1986 census. In terms of therapies utilized, 31 percent sought naturopathy, 39 percent homoeopathy, 36 percent herbalism, eleven percent remedial therapy/massage, six percent chiropractic or osteopathy, one percent acupuncture, and two percent didn't know or were not sure what kind of therapy they were seeking (Lloyd et al., 1993:139).

MacLennan, Wilson, and Taylor (1996) conducted what has become a classic baseline study of complementary medicine utilization in Australia.

They interviewed 3004 individuals over 15 years of age in what they describe as a representative sample of South Australians. They found that 48.5 percent of their interviewees were utilizing natural products and that 20.3 percent of their interviewees had visited at least one complementary practitioner in the past year, most commonly a chiropractor. The researchers reported that users of complementary medicine tended to be female, relatively young, employed, highly educated, and generally fit but consumed alcohol at a risk level. MacLennan et al. (1996:569) extrapolated that the Australian population spent $AU621 million Australian on natural products and therapists of $AU309 million on patient visits to complementary practitioners in 1993.

Begbie et al. (1996) conducted a survey of among cancer patients in public hospital oncology units, namely the specialist consulting rooms at the Royal North Shore Hospital and the Oncology Outpatient Clinic at Port Macquarie Base Hospital. Of the 507 patients visiting these clinics, 335 (66 percent) returned questionnaires, of which 319 (62 percent) were sufficiently complete. The survey indicated that 21.9 percent of the patients had utilised complementary therapies for cancer. Use of alternative therapies was associated with younger age and being married and negatively associated with satisfaction with conventional treatment. Forty percent of the respondents had not discussed their use of complementary therapies with their biomedical physicians.

McGregor and Peay (1996) conducted a study based upon telephone interviews in which they compared a sample of 81 patients (18 male and 67 female) at an alternative clinic near an Australian capital city with a community sample consisting of 81 respondents (25 male and 56 female). The 'Touch for Health' therapeutic system entailed 'techniques which have been developed with modern practice of ancient disciplines and knowledge in Oriental health management' (quoted in McGregor & Peay, 1996:1319). 'The two groups did not differ significantly on any of the demographic variables: gender, age, marital status, SES level of suburb, education, or occupation' (McGregor & Peay, 1996:1319). Furthermore, the researchers did not find any in significant difference between the two groups in term of the incidence of a chronic condition (McGregor & Peay, 1996:1323). They however, found that,

> For the alternative therapy group as a whole, the use of alternative therapies is associated with lack of trust in conventional medicine but also with 'unconventionality'… Those who use alternative therapies for functional reasons may also be more eclectic, patronising different therapy systems for different problems, and hence the association

of symptom treatment preference for alternative therapies with distrust of conventional medicine emerges in the preference for alternative therapies as a whole rather than a particular regime (McGregor &
Peay, 1996:1325).

Bensoussan and Myers (1996:123–131) distributed a survey to two groups
of practitioners: (1) 100 non-biomedical Traditional Chinese Medicine practitioners randomly selected from a database of all Traditional Chinese Medicine
practitioners in Victoria, New South Wales, and Queensland derived from a
University of Western Sydney (UWSM) mailing list; and (2) 100 biomedical
physicians who practice Traditional Chinese Medicine, primarily acupuncture, randomly selected from a combined mailing list created by Australian
Medical Acupuncture Society (AMAS) in conjunction with the Integrative
Medicine Association and Australian Chinese Medical Association. They asked
the practitioners to request each patient treated on a specific clinic day to
complete the survey. A total of 274 completed patient contact forms were
received from the 59 responding practitioners (33 from the UWSM mailing
list and 26 from AMAS mailing list). The response rate from UWSM list was
46 percent and from the AMAS list 26 percent. Of the 51 completed forms
from the patients of biomedical TCM practitioners and 223 from patients
of the primary non-biomedical practitioners, approximately two thirds of
the patients were female (Bensoussan & Myers, 1996). Approximately
55 percent of the patients who saw TCM practitioners had been educated
in tertiary institutions, including technical and private colleges, as opposed
to 18 percent of the patients who had obtained treatment from biomedical
physicians. Eighty-three percent of the patients listed English as their first
language whereas seven percent listed Chinese or another Asian language as
their first language. While patients' occupation was identified in only about
half of the responses, of those that were, 39 percent were in managerial or
professional sectors. Only 33 percent of all the patients carried private health
insurance that covered TCM treatment. Of those seeing non-biomedical
TCM practitioners, 63 percent carried no insurance for this treatment, while
78 percent of those who saw biomedical physicians did not carry private
health insurance, but were eligible for coverage under Medicare.

Kerrode, Myers, and Ramsey (1999) conducted a telephone survey that
sought to identify users of complementary therapies on the North Coast
of New South Wales. They had a response rate of 44 percent. Out of 645
respondents, 434 reported that they utilized complementary therapies.
Sixty-nine percent of the users of complementary therapies were women
(Kermode et al., 1999:15). There was no appreciable difference between
users and non-users of complementary therapies with respect to income
level or subscription to private health insurance. Twelve percent of the users

were above the national average in terms of income, 20 percent were at about the national average, and 68 percent below the national average. Conversely the users exhibited a slightly higher level of education overall than the non-users. Fifty percent of the users had visited chiropractors or osteopaths, whereas 35 percent had seen naturopaths and 35 percent massage thera-pists. Females were more likely to see naturopaths than males were. Users of complementary therapies also saw acupuncturists/TCM practitioners, herbalists, homeopaths, and counsellors or psychologists.

While patient utilization of complementary medicine tends to be associ-ated with urban areas, some rural areas or country towns depending upon their demographics may exhibit a high level of patient utilization. A case in point is a survey conducted by Sherwood (2000) of 268 people, 30 percent of whom are residents of Bunbury, 19 percent of Busselton, 6 percent of Dunsborough, 20 percent of Margaret River, and 25 percent in the rural hinterlands of these coastal shires of the south-western region of Western Australia. Respondents were randomly chosen in street surveys during 1995, 177 (66 percent) of whom were female and 91 (34 percent) of whom were male. In terms of occupation, '17 percent (45) described themselves as professionals, 15 percent (41) full-time parents, 13 percent (35) students, 12 percent (33) in the trades, 9 percent (25) retired, 8 percent (21) cleri-cal workers, 7 percent (19) in retail, 5 percent (12) in the service indus-try, 5 percent (12) unemployed and 9 percent (12) other' (Sherwood, 2000:195). While 51 percent of the respondents had used some sort of complementary practitioner in the previous years, Sherwood does not indi-cate which occupational groups were more or less like to do so. She does note, however, that the area attracts alternative life-stylers, youth, and 'rural resettlers' (many of whom are professionals), and retirees. It very likely that the first and third of these social categories would be particularly drawn to complementary medicine.

Wilkinson (2001) conducted an extensive survey in the Riverina section of New South Wales that drew upon 314 completed questionnaires out of 1000 mailed questionnaires. Respondents were asked which natural products they had used and complementary therapists they had seen during the previ-ous year, about their attitudes toward complementary medicine, the sources of their information about it, and which ailments they had. Respondents were 64.8 percent female, had a median age of 45, married in 72.3 percent of cases, and retired in 33.3 percent of cases. 32.7 percent of the respon-dents occupied blue collar and technical positions whereas 21 percent occu-pied white-collar positions. Wilkinson (2001) found that 70.3 percent of the respondents had utilized complementary therapies and 62.7 percent of them had a seen a complementary therapist. Chiropractic had been utilized by 26.1 percent of the respondents and massage therapy by 25.1 percent of them. Whereas females were more inclined to use vitamin and mineral therapy, herbal medicine, and aromatherapy and see herbalists, traditional Chinese practitioners, homeopaths, and iridologists, men were more likely to rely upon chiropractors. Respondents obtained information about complementary therapies from friends (64.5 percent of cases), the internet (3.2 percent of cases), other health practitioners (3.65 percent), newspapers (22.2 percent of cases), and TV/radio (22.2 percent of cases). In terms of attitudes toward complementary therapies, 56.2 percent believed that they had improved their health, 43.8 percent believed they were of limited use, and 53.4 percent believed that they provided a meaningful alternative when biomedical treatments had failed.

Adams, Sibbritt, Easthope, and Young (2003) conducted a cross-sectional postal questionnaire in 1996 drawing upon a baseline survey of the Australian Longitudinal Study on Women's Health that included over 40,000 Australian women consisting of samples from three age cohorts and urban and non-urban areas. The survey found that complementary medicine users were more likely to be older, resided proportionately in non-urban areas more than in urban areas, reported poorer health, and exhibited more symptoms and illnesses, and relied more on biomedical services than non-users. Twenty-eight percent of the women in the mid-age cohort consulted a complementary therapist in the previous year whereas only 19 percent in the younger cohort and 15 percent in the older cohort did so.

Based upon interview and focus group research in Oceanport (pseudonym), a socio-economically diverse suburb of a New South Wales city, anthropologist Linda Connor (2004) found that 27 (24 percent) of her 111 subjects indicated that they or another household member had engaged in a pattern of 'mixed therapy regimens' – a scenario in which 'people may be using multiple types of therapists and therapies simultaneously, or shift from one type of therapy or practitioner to another in seeking to solve their health problems. Other studies also indicate that most patients who rely on complementary medicine also continue to utilize biomedicine (D'Crus & Wilkinson, 2005).

In contrast to various studies that draw upon regional or local populations, Xue, Zhang, Lin, Da Costa, and Story (2007) conducted a national study of the utilisation of complementary medicine in Australia. During May–June 2005, they interviewed 1067 adults from all Australian states and territories which they recruited by random-digit telephone dialling. In a twelve month period, more than nine percent (68) of their interviewees responded having utilised at least one of 17 forms of complementary medicine and 44.1 percent visited a complementary practitioner. According to Xue et al.,

> The estimated number of visits to CAM [complementary and alternative medicine] practitioners by adult Australians in the 12-month period (69.2) was almost identical to the estimate number of visits to medical practitioners (69.3 million). The annual 'out of pocket' expenditure on CAM, nationally, was estimated as 4.13 billion Australian dollars (US $3.12 billion). Less than half of the users informed their medical practitioners about their use of CAM. The most common characteristics of CAM users were: age, 18–34; female; employed; well-educated; private health insurance coverage; and higher-than-average incomes (Xue et al., 2007:643).

In terms of the utilisation of special types of complementary medicine, 45.8 percent had used clinical nutrition, 27.2 Western massage therapy, 17.5 percent meditation, 16.3 percent Western herbal medicine, 16.1 percent aromatherapy, 16.1 percent chiropractic, 12.0 percent yoga, 10.7 naturopathy, 9.2 percent acupuncture, 7.0 percent Chinese herbal medicine, 7.0 percent energy healing, 6.0 percent homeopathy, 6.0 percent *qigong*, martial arts, and *t'ai chi*, 5.1 percent Chinese therapeutic massage, 4.6 percent osteopathy, 4.1 percent reflexology, and 2.3 percent Chinese medicine dietary therapy (Xue et al., 2007:646).

The Australian government's 2004–2005 Health Survey indicated that in 2004–2005, 32 percent of the Australian population (6.4 million people) had consulted a biomedical physician, dentist, chemist, or a biomedical-type practitioner, such as a physiotherapist, psychologist, or audiologist during the previous two weeks (Australian Bureau of Statistics, 2008:3). In contrast,

> 3.8 percent of the population (748,000 people) had consulted one of seven selected complementary health therapists [chiropractors, naturopaths, acupuncturists, osteopaths, herbalists, traditional healers, and hypnotherapists] in the previous two weeks... The most commonly consulted were chiropractors (433,000 visitors), naturopaths (134,000 visitors) and acupuncturists (96,000 visitors) (Australian Bureau of Statistics, 2008:3).

Various social scientists have sought to explain reasons that so many people, particularly upper and upper-middle class ones, have turned to complementary medicine in developed countries, such as the United States and the United Kingdom. A group of sociologists and health researchers have also drawn attention to this issue in Australia (Siahpush, 1999). While a review of studies on patient utilization of complementary medicine in Australia indicates various patterns, overall these studies indicate that like other Western societies users of complementary medicine tend to be female, relatively young, employed, highly educated, and often, but not necessarily generally, involved in alternative lifestyles. Conversely, complementary medicine has found some reception among working-class Australians, including ones living in country towns. The evidence demonstrates that many Australians have turned to chiropractic, osteopathy, acupuncture and Chinese herbal medicine, naturopathy or natural therapies, homeopathy, vitamin and nutritional supplements, and an array of lesser-known therapeutic systems, such as Reiki, iridology, reflexology, and aromatherapy. By and large, however, it appears that the primary consumers of complementary medicine in Australia are relatively affluent individuals who can afford to pay for it either out of pocket or have part of their expenses covered under a private health plan. Most of the some 43 registered private health plans 'refund a proportion of professional fees incurred for chiropractic and osteopathy, while professional fees for acupuncture, naturopathy, homoeopathy and remedial massage are covered by many funds' (Weir, 2005:36). Conversely, only a few health funds provide coverage for modalities such as kinesiology, iridology and Alexander Technique (Weir, 2005:36).

Siahpush empirically tested three common theories that seek to explain why complementary medicine has grown in popularity – namely, dissatisfaction with the health outcomes of biomedicine, dissatisfaction with the biomedical encounter, and the emergence of a postmodern value system. He conducted structured interviews based upon a 'telephone survey of 209 non-institutionalised adult residents in the 060 area code in Australia (Albury-Wodonga region, north east Victoria and an adjacent area in New South Wales)' in which only 11.5 percent of the potential informants refused to participate (Siahpush, 1998:62). Statistical analysis of the responses in the survey led Siahpush (1998:67) to conclude 'that the latter two hypotheses hold ground and that the emergence of postmodern values, compared to dissatisfaction with the medical encounter, provides a better explanation for the popularity of alternative medicine'. He maintains that the growing popularity of green culture, natural foods, and consumerism and growing awareness of the health hazards of modern technology have been prompting many people to turn to complementary therapies (Siahpush, 1998:68). In a somewhat similar vein, Rayner and Easthope (2001:174) argue that the consumption of natural medicine products illustrates the presence of 'niche markets delineated by life style, an emphasis on symbolic value rather than use value and the use of such medicines as a means of self-assembly – all features predicted by theorists of postmodern society'.

Gary Easthope (2005:338–342) delineates five theories that have been proposed for the growing popularity of complementary medicine: (1) the search for explaining the meaning of illness other than the germ theory associated with biomedicine, such as 'in terms of spiritual forces (spiritualism), the balance of elements in the body (yin and yang, naturopathy), or the development of life force (homoeopathy)'; (2) an increased distrust of scientific experts associated with biomedicine; (3) a more 'personal' healer–patient relationship associated with many complementary medical systems; (4) the search for increased personal control in what many scholars have term 'postmodern' societies; and (5) a growing concern in treating chronic and terminal diseases as infectious diseases have come under control, at least in developed societies. Various other studies also posit that the utilization of complementary therapies is part and parcel of the adoption of post-modern values, particularly among those who enjoy the luxury of participating in a culture of consumption (O'Callaghan & Jordon, 2003).

Summary

Many complementary medical systems, particularly naturopathy, Western herbalism, Chinese medicine, and homeopathy, and bodywork, underwent rejuvenation within the context of the holistic health movement and continue to thrive as numerous patient utilisation studies have indicated. In addition to professionalised or partially-professionalised heterodox medical systems, religious healing systems and folk medical systems of various forms constitute important components of Australian medical pluralism. In that professionalised and partially-professionalised complementary systems are not covered under Medicare and require out-of-pocket payments or partial payment through private health plans, they tend to be out of the financial reach of many lower-middle class, working class, and poor Australians. As a consequence, complementary medicine has in large part become domain of the more affluent sectors of Australian society. Conversely, it is very likely that many of the less affluent people in Australia, particularly those belonging to various ethnic minorities, employ a variety of religious and folk healing traditions.

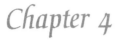

Chapter 4

Government inquiries and statutory recognition of complementary medical practices

Introduction

Statutes in New South Wales, South Australia, Western Australia, Tasmania, and the Northern Territory stipulate that only biomedical physicians can 'practice medicine' (Weir, 2000b:27). Conversely, Queensland and Victoria do not prohibit biomedical practice by unregistered individuals. Aside from chiropractors and osteopaths who hold statutory registration in all Australian states and territories – and acupuncturists and Traditional Chinese Medicine practitioners who obtained statutory recognition in Victoria in 2000 – all other complementary medicine practitioners have to date not obtained statutory registration elsewhere in Australia, even though many of them would like to have it. Many complementary medicine practitioners deny that they diagnose lest they be charged with 'practicing medicine' (Weir, 2000b:29). Conversely, complementary medicine practitioners are regarded to constitute 'health service providers in health rights complaints legislation in all states and territories except South Australia' (Weir, 2000b:32). Some complementary medicine groups have not been able to create a self-regulatory system that has broad support of its various associations and practitioners (Carlton & Bensoussan, 2002:22). This situation permits practitioners with minimal or no formal training to establish clinics and use the titles of a particular complementary medicine group.

The Webb Report of 1977 conflates 'naturopathy' and 'natural therapy' and argues that inquiries in New South Wales, Victoria, and at the federal level prompted a loose assemblage of naturopaths or natural therapists to amalgamate the South Pacific Federation of Natural Therapeutics and the Australian Council for Natural Therapies into the South Pacific Council for Natural Therapies in July 1975 (Committee of Inquiry, 1977). The Committee was critical of the courses offered at naturopathic or natural therapy colleges and asserted that while the syllabi of many of these institutions 'were reasonable in their coverage of basic biomedical sciences on paper, the actual instruction bore little relationship to the documented course'.

Since the Webb Report, the federal government and various state governments have conducted inquiries into both complementary practitioners and complementary medicines. State and territory governments have tended to encourage most complementary medicine associations to create self-regulatory registrations. All states and territories have laws that restrict prescribing and dispensing of certain herbs that contain substances that are deemed potentially dangerous. These laws have prevented complementary practitioners from 'legally using some of the tools of their trade' (Carlton & Bensoussan, 2002:21). Carlton and Bensoussan (2002:21) assert that '[a]s a consequence, illegal prescribing of some of these herbs is widespread amongst practitioners'.

The road to the statutory recognition for Chinese medicine and acupuncture in victoria

Prior to 2000 Chinese medicine practitioners and acupuncturists in Australia had been unable to create a self-regulatory registration system that received the broad support of the majority of associations and practitioners (Carlton & Bensoussan, 2002:22). The National Health and Medical Research Council (NHMRC), a federal body that plays a key role in medical research, first investigated acupuncture in 1974 and simply rejected as having no place in medicine (Beer, 2005:233). In 1987 NHMRC appointed a working group to investigate acupuncture which concluded that acupuncture should fall under biomedical care. O'Neill (1994a:100–101), who obtained access to the working party's papers under the Freedom of Information Act, maintains that the proceedings of the working group contained a strong biomedical bias in that practitioners affiliated with the Australian Acupuncture College in Melbourne were unfairly associated with a death ten years earlier following treatment by an acupuncturist. The Australian Medical Acupuncture Society – an association representing biomedical physicians who perform acupuncture – had privileged access to the working group. Furthermore, although 'submissions were invited and obtained from traditional acupuncture organizations, the working group did not inspect private colleges and relied on damaging generalisations about their staff, students and courses by medical practitioners who had not visited them either' (O'Neill, 1994a:101). Ultimately the working group recommended that the practice of acupuncture be restricted to biomedical physicians.

Subsequently, the Acupuncture Ethics and Standards Organization (AESO) and the acupuncture colleges obtained a meeting with the chairperson of the NHMRC health care committee (O'Neill, 1994a:117). They requested formation of another working group that would identify the role and place of acupuncture in health care system. The NHMRC responded by creating a Working Party on the Role and Requirements for Acupuncture Education (O'Neill, 1994a:119). The working party defined acupuncture as a primary care modality and recommended that acupuncture education be situated in tertiary education as well as postgraduate training for other health professionals interested in practising acupuncture. The Australian Acupuncture College in Melbourne began a drive to recruit students in anticipation of possible absorption of its program of study by La Trobe University, a development that never came to fruition (O'Neill, 1994a:120).

In October 1995 the Victorian Department of Human Services solicited tenders for research to assess the benefits and risks associated with Chinese Medicine, survey the nature of Chinese medicine workforce in Victoria, and the need for legislative regulation of Chinese medicine in Victoria in October 1995 (Benssousan & Myers, 1996:1). The Health Departments of New South Wales and Queensland joined the review with the intention of broadening the study to include their states. In November 1996, the project report, which was based on collaborative research between the Victoria Department of Health Services, Southern Cross University, and the University of Western Sydney, was issued (Bensoussan & Myers, 1996). The AHMAC endorsed the Working Group's recommendations that Chinese medicine and acupuncture be granted statutory registration.

The Australian Health Ministers Advisory Council (AHMAC, est. 1995) has established processes and criteria for assessing applications for registration from unregistered health occupations. It consists of the heads of all State and Commonwealth Health Departments and has the responsibility for making recommendations to State, Territory and Federal Health Ministers on matters of common concern. The Council has a policy that stipulates that 'no health occupation will be registered by any state without agreement from the majority of states' (quoted in *Review of Traditional Chinese Medicine, Newsletter No. 3, March 1998 (Summary)*). It endorsed the Victorian review process in February 1997 and stipulated that Victoria take the lead in developing a proposal for regulation of Chinese medicine and acupuncture.

Despite opposition from Australian Medical Acupuncture Society, the Australasian Integrated Medical Association, the Australian College of Physical Medicine, the Australian College of Herbal Medicine, and the Royal Australian College of General Practitioners, the Victorian Parliament passed the Chinese Medicine Registration Act in May 2000, making Victoria the only Australian jurisdiction to formally regulate TCM practitioners. The Act requires Chinese medicine practitioners to use title 'acupuncturist', 'Chinese herbal medicine practitioner', or 'Chinese medicine practitioner', and to register with the Chinese Medicine Registration Board. This body consists of,

> Nine members nominated by the Minister [of Health] and appointed by Governor in Council. The members will be comprised of six registered practitioners, a lawyer and two persons not registered practitioners. At least two members of the board must be able to communicate in English and either Mandarin or any other Chinese dialect (Weir, 2000b:152). Although a small number of complementary medicine associations initially opposed statutory recognition of acupuncture and Chinese medicine in Victoria, reportedly 'most have since changed their position and now support registration' (Carlton & Bensoussan, 2002:25). Seven hundred forty practitioners have been registered under the Act (Lin, 2004:96). Although the Chinese Registration Board of Victoria accepted Advanced Diplomas until December 2007, for applicants after this date it requires a minimum of a Bachelor Degree.

Part and parcel of the process of the legitimation of Chinese medicine and acupuncture has been governmental recognition of Chinese medicine training programs in private schools and governmental support of Chinese medicine training programs in public universities. The Sydney acupuncture college obtained accreditation from the state of New South Wales with assistance from a public tertiary institution (O'Neill, 1994a:104). Conversely, when the Melbourne acupuncture college, which had contracted for the teaching of biomedical science courses at the Lincoln Institute of Health Sciences, submitted a proposal to develop an undergraduate degree program at the institution, the physiotherapy staff at Lincoln opposed the plan by arguing that only biomedical physicians, veterinarians, and dentists possess the knowledge to apply acupuncture safely (O'Neill, 1994a:106). The possibility of creating an acupuncture program at Lincoln died with latter's absorption into La Trobe University. The acupuncture colleges and AESO responded by establishing the Australian Council on Acupuncture and Traditional Chinese Medical Education (O'Neill, 1994a:113). Conversely, the traditional acupuncture groups opposed ACATCME which they viewed as front organization for colleges. The AESO and colleges widened their campaign against the NHMRC (Bensoussan & Myers, 1996).

Eventually, as is noted in greater detail in the following chapter, Chinese medicine programs came to be offered at three public universities, namely the Royal Melbourne of Technology University (RMIT), University of Technology, Sydney, the Victoria University of Technology. Australian Acupuncture College in Sydney became part of the University of Technology, Sydney that offers the Bachelor of Applied Science (Acupuncture) (Jacka, 1998:160). The Victoria University of Technology absorbed the sister course in Melbourne in

1992 and offers a Bachelor Degree in Health Science (Acupuncture). RMIT University developed a Master's degree in acupuncture.

Although there are numerous training programs in acupuncture and Chinese medicine and acupuncture, AACMA restricts its 'recognised course list' to those at four public universities, namely the University of Technology, Sydney, the University of Western Sydney, the Royal Institute of Technology, and Victoria University of Technology, and only three private colleges, namely Sydney Institute of Traditional Chinese Medicine, the Australian College of Traditional Medicine in Queensland, and the Melbourne College of Traditional Medicine. Whereas most of the membership of AACMA consists of European Australians, the leadership and membership of the Chinese Health Foundation of Australia appears to consist of Asians, particularly of Chinese extraction (Chinese Health Foundation of Australia, hom.vicnet. net.au, accessed 20/7/2008). The Australian Chinese Medicine Education & Research Council (est. 1995) focuses on the academic development of Chinese medicine in Australia (mc2.vicnet.au, accessed 20/07/2008). Fifteen acupuncture and Chinese medicine associations along with the Australian Traditional Medicine Society and Australian Natural Therapists Association collaborated in the creation of national educational guidelines with the aim of achieving statutory in other political jurisdictions other than Victoria, but to date this effort has not resulted in such an achievement (National Academic Standards Committee for Traditional Chinese Medicine, 2001).

Only time will tell whether Chinese medicine will achieves statutory registration in other Australian jurisdictions. The Western Australian Department of Health (2005) released a report which suggests various criteria that could be employed in the possible implementation of statutory registration for Chinese medicine practitioners in Western Australia. The Australian Traditional Medicine Society (2005) quickly responded to this report in which it admitted several advantages of statutory registration but drew up a longer listing of disadvantages. As a consequence, ATMS recommends the implementation of a system of co-regulation in which TCM training programs would be accredited by the Western Australian government but a Chinese medicine professional association would regulate practitioners. Somewhat later a New South Wales parliamentary committee has explored the possibility of statutory registration for Chinese medicine practitioners (Committee on the Health Care Complaints Commission, 2005).

The widespread presence of Chinese medicine clinics in Australian capital cities, regional cities, and even country towns testifies to the wide-spread public acceptance of Chinese medicine. Conversely, to some extent, as is demonstrated later in this book, biomedicine has been co-opting the foremost modality of Chinese medicine, namely acupuncture. Tiqua (2004:269), a Chinese medicine practitioner, argues that biomedicalisation has reduced acupuncture into a simple procedure which has become 'stripped of its vitalist philosophical core – the philosophy of Qi'. Despite this, in his capacity as traditional Chinese practitioner, he was permitted to administer acupuncture to a 70 year old woman at the Austin hospital (Tiqua, 2004:317).

Whereas chiropractors and osteopaths now receive limited reimbursements for Medicare for services rendered, this does not apply to Chinese medicine practitioners in the one political jurisdiction – Victoria – where they enjoy statutory registration. Conversely, biomedical physicians are reimbursed under Medicare for rendering acupuncture.

The drive for statutory recognition by natural therapists and other complementary practitioners

In contrast to chiropractors and osteopaths and Chinese medicine practitioners in Victoria, statutory registration has been a matter that has eluded naturopaths and other natural therapists in Australia. Natural therapists enjoyed statutory registration for several years in the sparely-populated Northern Territory beginning in 1985 when the legislative assembly passed the Allied Health and Professional Practitioners Act. The naturopathic section of the Act was based on the curriculum of the Southern School of Naturopathy and granted registration only to members of the Australian National Therapists Association (Jacka, 1998:124). However, efforts to implement statutory registration for natural therapists in both the New South Wales and Victoria around the same time failed.

The Social Development Committee (1986:v) commissioned by the Parliament of Victoria recommended that natural therapists should not be registered, despite its recognition that complementary medicine plays a 'very significant role in the life of many Victorians'. The Committee entertained the views of several natural therapy associations, particularly the Australian Natural Therapists Association and the Australian Traditional Medicine Society. Whereas the former favoured statutory registration and the establishment of single colleges of complementary medicine with a strong emphasis on the basic sciences in each state, the latter, which claimed to represent some 16 complementary colleges and their alumni and students, opposed statutory registration and viewed the ANTA approach as an effort to create a monopoly (Social Development Committee, 1986:170). While the ATMS has questioned the relevance of biomedical science in the teaching of the natural therapies, it did plan to incorporate the basic health sciences into the curricula of its member colleges (Social Development Committee, 1986:140). The Social Development Committee strongly recommended that government require practising natural therapists to complete biomedical sciences courses. The Australian Naturopathic Practitioners and Chiropractors Association, a small Victorian body, also favoured statutory registration of natural therapists but the Acupuncture Ethics and Standards Organisation argued for a separate system of statutory registration for acupuncturists (Social Development Committee, 1986:171–172). Representatives of the Orthomolecular Medical Association of Australia (a branch of biomedicine that advocates the integration of nutritional and alternative therapies) also provided input to the Committee (Social Development Committee, 1986:74).

Most recently the Victorian Department of Health Services commissioned the School of Public Health at La Trobe University to conduct a study of the benefits, risks, and the possible merits of statutory regulation pertaining to naturopathy and Western herbal medicine (Lin et al., 2005). The study team recognises that 'herbal medicine is a core practice for naturopaths' and recommended the regulation of both naturopathy and Western herbal medicine given that both of them entail potential risk to the public (Lin et al., 2005:14). In a national survey of general practitioners, the study team found that 77 percent of them favoured the regulation of various complementary medicine practitioner occupations: 'In relation to specific therapies, GPs strongly supported regulation for acupuncture (87 percent of respondents), Chinese herbal medicine (80 percent), herbal medicine (77 percent), naturopathy (73 percent), homeopathy (66 percent), and vitamin and mineral therapy (66 percent)' (Lin et al., 2005:11).

The federal government adopted a policy of mutual recognition of statutory registration that 'meant that there was to be uniformity between states and it was no longer acceptable to have registration for a profession in one state and not in another'. This policy coupled with an objection from the Australian Traditional-Medicine Society that its members were not eligible for statutory registration resulted in the Northern Territory Legislative Territory withdrawing this privilege for natural therapists in general (personal communication with Sue Evans, Lecturer, School of Natural and Complementary Medicine, Southern Cross University, 4 November 2004).

As this incident suggests, a major factor that has prevented many complementary practitioners, particularly natural therapists but also practitioners of Traditional Chinese Medicine outside of Victoria, to obtain statutory registration in the various jurisdictions of Australia is that they are divided into numerous associations. Table 7 depicts a partial listing of natural therapies associations in existence at the present time in Australia. President Bill Pearson (2002:158) noted in his address at the Australian Traditional-Medicine Society Annual General Meeting in Melbourne on 22 September 2002 the existence of 43 complementary associations in Australia and that ATMS represents 31 different modalities.

The Australian Natural Therapists Association (est. 1955) developed from an amalgamation of several groups of which the most significant were

Table 7
A partial listing
of natural
therapies
associations in
Australia

Association	Year established
National Herbalists Association of Australia	1921
Australian Natural Therapies Association	1955
Australian Council of Natural Therapies	1974
Australian Naturopathic Practitioners Association	1975
Australian Traditional-Medicine Society	1984
Federation of Natural & Traditional Therapists	1991
Alumni Association of Natural Medicine Practitioners	1992
Australasian Federation of Natural Therapists	1996

the National Association of Naturopaths and the Australian Chiropractors, Osteopaths, and Naturopathic Physicians Association (Jacka, 1998:81). It reportedly constitutes the second largest natural therapies association in Australia (ANTA, 2004:2). ANTA is governed by a National Council or Board of Directors who are elected by the members for three years and has a National Remedial Therapy Chairperson, a National Naturopathy Chairperson, and a National Homoeopathy Chairperson. It also claims to represent nutritionists, herbalists, Chinese medicine practitioners, acupuncturists, osteopaths, chiropractors, Ayurvedic practitioners, and aramotherapists, and lists over fifty private health funds that recognize its practitioners for provider status (www.anta.com.au, accessed 26/1/2008).

Dorothy Hall, an herbalist, founded the Australian Traditional-Medicine Society in 1984 (Martyr, 2002:278). ATMS is the largest single natural therapies association in Australia and consists of departments of massage therapy, Traditional Chinese Medicine, homoeopathy, naturopathic nutrition, naturopathy, and Western herbal medicine (www.atms.com.au/body.htm). It claimed in July 2006 to have had 10,601 'financial members' (www.atms.com.au, accessed 17/02/2009).

ATMS is governed by the owners of various private ATMS-accredited colleges and does not permit its rank-and-file members to vote for board members and members of various working committees. Dorothy Hall (1998:119) defends this pattern of bureaucratic centralism in the following way,

> As a newly ATMS Accredited member, did you know enough about anyone it to form an opinion of whether they would have the capability to be Director? But you did have the knowledge of the ATMS college that trained you. You did know who ran that, and how long it had been in business, and what its teaching programs were like, its student information, etc. So, to me, this seemed the logical place to supply the positions of ATMS Directors, those who had already proved their competence and gained their experience over many years. From the

colleges we should be able to blend joint wisdom, hard earned over time, and form the ATMS 'Cabinet' (Hall, 1998:119).

She encourages the members to attend the annual general meeting, which is held away Sydney every other year, where they will have the 'opportunity to meet Executives, ask questions, hear our reports of how we have looked after you and socialises' (Hall, 1998:20). ATMS claims to represent 65 percent of complementary practitioners in Australia. Its membership has grown from 3200 members in 1994 to 9550 in 2004 and claims to represent '39 full accredited colleges, plus another 40 provisionally acted' (Easthope, 2005:326).

The National Herbalists Association of Australia has been publishing the *Australian Journal of Medical Herbalism* since 1989. Its has been lobbying for statutory registrations for Western herbalism and its membership includes many naturopaths. NHAA has four active state chapters: the VicHerbs Chapter, the Queensland Chapter, the South Australia State Chapter, and the WA [Western Australia] State Chapter.

I had the opportunity to attend several sessions and other events at the Fifth International Conference on Phytotherapeutics sponsored by NHAA on 19 March 2004 in Canberra. At the opening session, Susan Dean, the NHAA President addressed an audience of 300–400 practitioners, students, and visitors, perhaps 75–80 percent of whom were women. The dress attire of the attendees tended to be relatively casual, and even semi-bohemian or alternative on the part of many of them. Dean noted that a multitude of bodies represent herbalists and naturopaths in Australia and that NHAA has been promoting a self-regulatory model for its membership. She noted that members should view governmental studies of complementary practices, educational standards, and natural products as an opportunity to achieve greater legitimacy in the larger society. Dean added that herbalists want to ensure that they offer safe and efficacious medicines. She noted that various speakers at the conference will help practitioners in developing their clinical skills. Dean introduced the NHAA board to the audience, which consisted of eight women and two men.

Kakkib li'Dthia Warrawee'a, a short balding, stocky man with a beard and wearing his hair in a pony tail and of mixed Aboriginal and European ancestry, presented the opening keynote address titled 'Where is the Wisdom We have Lost in Knowledge?' in the early afternoon. He identified himself as a 'traditional Aboriginal medicine man', a 'doctor of a holistic way', and the author of *There Once Was a Tree Called Deru*. Kakkib waved a boomerang periodically during the course of his talk. One of my informants told me that he had carried a big stick at another conference which she had attended.

Kakkib alluded to the technology of the 'white fellahs' and said a prayer to the Aboriginal ancestors while holding a long feather. He told the audience that he had been trained as a spiritual teacher since birth when his people chanted to him. Kakkib told the audience,

> You want to hear that this herb is used for what. This is my country. The Ya-idt'midung are my people. We have between 260 and 700 Aboriginal medicines. We have as many medicines as we have nations… Culture plays an enormous role in medicine. We got buggards of information coming out of our ears. In medicine today we have become more informed but less wise. This is true for both allopathic medicine and complementary and alternative medicine… We practiced preventative medicine. Preventive medicine could be called holistic. What is this thing 'holistic'? Mind-body-spirit? Right, wrong. Environment plays an enormous role…. All this paper and technology drives a bloke crazy.

Kakkib showed the audience a slide depicting Abraham Maslow's hierarchy of needs and noted that Maslow was wrong and stated,

> First and foremost is that we have a reason to live… Many Aboriginal People have lost a reason to live… What is spirituality? It is not the same as religion. Truth is inside of you… Traditional Aboriginal medicine is not herbal medicine… How many of you consider your patients' social, environmental, and spiritual condition?

In a session titled 'Regulation of CM Professions – Where are We going?', Anne-Louisie Carlston, a Senior Policy Analyst in the Policy and Strategic Projects Division of the Victorian Department of Social Services' delineated various models for the regulation of professions. She noted that the track record of self-regulation has not been good due to professional and personal rivalries among complementary medicine bodies, a lack of consensus on practice standards, and a lack of commitment to self-regulation. Carlston described the Chinese Medical Regulatory Board structure in Victoria and noted that the vast majority of acupuncturists and practitioners of Chinese medicine in Victoria have opted to be registered. Some of the talks at the conference included 'Traditional Medicine within Tibetan Health' presented by a female naturopath from Melbourne, 'Food is More Than Nutrition: Cross-Cultural Uses of Chicken Soup' presented by another Melbourne female naturopath and a PhD student in medical anthropology.

I had the opportunity to attend the Sixth International Conference on Phytotherapeutics which convened on 21–23 September 2007. Along with Gerry Bodeker, a public health professor at Oxford University Medical School, I was one of observers of the complementary medicine scene to give presentations at the conference. Whereas Bodeker spoke about 'Global Trends in Natural Healthcare', I discussed 'The Growing Legitimation of Complementary Medicine in Australia'. Both of our presentations were enthusiastically received by the audience.

Natural therapists created an umbrella organization called the Natural Therapists Forum in 1991 'so that practitioners would continue to receive practitioner-only therapeutic goods and advertising material in accordance with the Therapeutic Goods Regulation' (Khoury, 1994:15). The Forum was renamed the Federation of Natural and Traditional Therapists and is made up of natural therapy associations. Other bodies that represent natural therapists and more specifically naturopaths include the Australian Council of Natural Therapies Education Australia, the Alumni Association of Natural Medicine Practitioners, and the Complementary Medicine Association.

Some associations consist of practitioners, consumers, natural products manufacturers, researchers, and natural therapists. The Australian Complementary Health Association (ACHA) represents practitioners and consumers and seeks to make 'complementary therapies more affordable, through rebates from health insurance schemes and Medicare, inclusion in workers compensation cover, and encouraging discounts for consumers' and calls for the inclusion of complementary therapies in hospitals, clinics, community health centres, and other health care settings (www.diversity.org.au/about.html, p. 4, accessed 29/03/2008). It publishes *Diversity: Natural & Complementary Health*. The National Health Care Alliance based in Cremorne, NSW, claims to function as a spokesperson for Australian natural health care industry manufacturers, distributors, sellers, educators, researchers and practitioners to the government and the public (www.nhca.com.au) (See Appendix 2 for more details on other natural therapy or complementary associations).

While the major natural therapy associations favour statutory registration and rigorous educational requirements for practitioners, another amorphous group of natural therapists opposes these elements. As Hunter (1991:3) observes, 'Their contention is that any movement towards establishing a more 'scientific basis for the practice of natural therapies (via improved standards which include a more scientific orientation) will not only exclude practitioners who have an intuitive rather than a scientific style of practice, but will ultimately lead to the erosion of the philosophy which established naturopathy as a unique profession'. She asserts that the professional associations in this group 'represent a wide spectrum of practitioners whose educational backgrounds vary from full-time professional courses to part-time public interest courses' (Hunter, 1991:3).

The Western Australian Department of Training and Employment – Strategic Services Division commissioned a private firm, Peter and Associates (2000) to conduct a survey of complementary medicine training programs in the state of Western Australia. The consulting firm identified 21 institutions that train complementary practitioners of seven 'natural therapy professional sector groupings', namely naturopathy, homeopathy, Chinese medicine, Chinese herbalism, Western herbalism, acupuncture, and massage therapy, in Western Australia (Peter & Associates, 2000:48). It reported that no universities in Western Australia were providing courses on complementary medicine and expressed concern about the quality of instruction in some of these training programs (Peter & Associates, 2000:77).

The Victorian Department of Human Services funded a feasibility study in 2001–2002 investigating the possible establishment of a complementary medicine research centre in Victoria (O'Brien, 2004:113). The Victorian government has followed suit by announcing support for the Australian Research Centre for Complementary and Alternative Medicine.

The drive on the part of various complementary medicine practitioners, particularly Chinese medicine practitioners and natural therapists, for exemption from the General Sales Tax for health services has prompted many of them to abide by the Australian government's call for self-regulation or a voluntary registration system. The Government had implemented a 10 percent General Service Tax (GST) for goods and services as part of its tax reform package in 2000, but stipulated that qualified herbalists, acupuncturists, and naturopaths would be GST-free if they met certain criteria. These practitioners were granted an exemption from charging GST for their consultations on the conditions that their professional associations developed – on the proviso these professions would have developed a national professional registration system by July 2003 (Australian Complementary Health Association, 2002:10). The federal government granted $500,000 to facilitate this process and divided the funds equally among five major professional associations, namely the Australian Acupuncture and Chinese Medicine Association, Australian Natural Therapists Association, the Australian Traditional-Medicine Association, the Federation of Natural & Traditional Therapists, and the National Herbalists Association of Australia. The NHAA and FNTT decided to collaborate on joint proposal under umbrella of Australian Council for Complementary Medicine. The ANTA and ATMS joined their efforts in developing a joint proposal of their own and the AACMA decided to develop its on proposal for TCM practitioners. Section 21 of the New Tax System (Goods and Services Tax Transition) Act 1999 created a established sunset clause to allow acupuncturists, herbalists and naturopaths to have GST free status until 30 June 2003 (Pearson & Khoury, 2003:39).

In order to deal with the fall-out from a scandal involving Pan Pharmaceutical, a major natural products manufacturer, the Australian government established an Expert Committee on Complementary Medicines in the Health System in May 2003 (Expert Committee on Complementary Medicines in the Health System, 2003). While the Committee focused primarily on the regulation of natural products, it also recommended a strengthening of training programs for complementary practitioners and increased funding for research on complementary medicine. The Expert Committee on Complementary Medicines in the Health System (2003:23–25) recommended that the various governments should develop a nationally consistent statutory registration system for complementary practitioners, training for all practitioners who prescribe or provide advise on the use of natural therapeutic products, and increased government funding for research on complementary medicines.

In recent years specific political parties have generally deferred from adopting policies on the socio-political status of complementary medicine. The Democrats somewhat took the lead in this area several years ago. Senator Lyn Allison, the Deputy Leader of Democrats, took a leading role in the drafting of a policy paper on complementary medicine. This policy paper argued that the,

> balance is wrong in current health policy. The current focus on expensive, high tech, high medication, acute care is at the expense of prevention, early intervention. This is a false dichotomy that drives up health costs and does not deliver optimum health.

The Democrats' Reform Agenda had proposed the creation of a National Centre for Complementary Medicine, increased hospital access for complementary therapists, and greater representation of the complementary medicine profession on government bodies. The Democrats advocated self-regulation rather than statutory registration for complementary practitioners beyond those who already have attained it, namely chiropractors and osteopaths and Chinese medicine practitioners in Victoria. The Australian Democrats held Forums on Complementary Medicine in Melbourne on 18 May 2004 and in Sydney on 20 May. Speakers included Bill Pearson (President of the Australian Traditional-Medicine Society), Stephen Myers (Director of the Australian Centre of Complementary Medicine, and David Briggs (a representative from the Therapeutic Goods Administration).

Summary

While chiropractic and osteopathy have achieved considerable governmental legitimation and have undergone a certain process of biomedicalisation, a wide array of other complementary medical systems still find themselves in ambiguous, if not downright marginal, status vis-à-vis the Australian state. Other than chiropractic and osteopathy, the only complementary medical system to have achieved statutory registration is Chinese medicine and acupuncture, and only in Victoria. While on-going suspicion about the scientific validity of various complementary medical systems may serve as an impediment to their ability to obtain statutory registration, some complementary professions, perhaps particularly naturopathy, are highly fragmented both in terms of their associations and training programs and definitions of what constitutes a qualified practitioner.

Chapter 5

Schools and public education funding

Introduction

Complementary medicine education has evolved into a massive industry embedded in various institutions throughout Australia. As indicated earlier, numerous programs offering qualifications in various natural therapies, including naturopathy, Western herbal medicine, Traditional Chinese Medicine and acupuncture, homoeopathy, massage therapy, and aromatherapy exist in both private colleges and, since the mid-1990s, in public tertiary institutions in Australia. Evans (2000b) delineates three educational models in natural therapeutics in Australia: (1) the private college model; (2) the university partnership model; and (3) the government-funded university model. Private natural therapy schools in the 1960s and 1970s often included chiropractic, osteopathy, and TCM along with naturopathy and homoeopathy in their programs of study (Hunter, 2002:43). With the establishment of chiropractic and osteopathic training programs at public universities beginning in the early 1980s, the natural therapy colleges dropped instruction in chiropractic and osteopathy. Hunter (2002:44) reports that an estimated 400 to 500 students graduate annually from private complementary medicine colleges each year (Hunter, 2002:44).

McCabe (2005b) has identified 43 programs or schools providing training in naturopathy and Western herbal medicine alone in Australia. She lists 47 campuses which offer some 104 courses in naturopathy and Western medicine (McCabe, 2005b:119). Thirty-two (68 percent) of the campuses are situated at private colleges, four (8.5 percent) at TAFE (Technical and Advanced Further Education) colleges, and eleven (23.5 percent) at universities (McCabe, 2005b:120).

Private colleges of complementary medicine

In addition to various chiropractic and osteopathic programs situated in public as well as other complementary medical programs in public universities and even TAFEs, Australia has a tremendously large number of private colleges of complementary medicine. The oldest of these is the Southern School of Natural Therapies in Melbourne which started out as the Victorian

Branch College of the Australian National Naturopathic Association (www.ssnt.vic.edu.au/ssntcourses.asp, accessed 4/3/2008). It offers the Bachelor of Health Science (Naturopathy) that entails four years of full-time study but allows students to pursue this degree on a part-time basis as well (SSNT Courses). It also offers an Advanced Diploma in Traditional Chinese Medicine and Bachelor of Health Sciences (Chinese Medicine), an Advanced Diploma in Myotherapy, an Introduction to Naturopathy Certificate, and evening and week-end courses on massage. SSNT operates a clinic staffed by fourth students in which a wide array of natural therapies are utilized, including 'iridology, herbal medicine, homoeopathy, flower essences, dietary advice, nutritional therapy, celloid therapy, relaxation massage and Traditional Chinese Medicine, including Chinese herbal medicine, acupuncture, moxibustion and cupping' (Student Clinic, www.ssnt.vic.edu.au/clinics.asp, accessed 4/03/2008).

The largest of the private complementary medicine colleges is what until very recently was called the Australian College of Natural Medicine with branches in Brisbane, Gold Coast, and Perth and with its affiliate, the Melbourne College of Natural Medicine with campuses in Melbourne City and Box Hill (*ACNM Course Guide, 2007*; www.canm.edu.au). It emerged out of what had been the Brisbane branch of Acupuncture Colleges (Australia) (Sherwood, 2004:224). It has offered bachelor degree programs since 1998, including the Bachelor of Health Science (Acupuncture) at the Brisbane and Melbourne campuses; the Bachelor of Health Science (Homeopathy) at the Brisbane and Melbourne campuses; and the Bachelor of Health Science (Naturopathy) at the Brisbane, Melbourne, and Perth campuses. ACNM has received accreditation for new bachelor degrees in nutritional medicine, Western herbal medicine, and musculoskeletal therapy. It also offers numerous courses at the certificate, diploma, and advanced diploma levels that are accredited through the Vocational Education and Training Authority. More specifically, ACNM offers advanced diplomas of acupuncture, homeopathy, naturopathy, nutritional medicine, and Western herbal medicine and diplomas of remedial massage, reflexology, aromatherapy, holistic counselling practices, and beauty therapy, and certificates in massage, TCM remedial massage, and beauty therapy. Its courses are recognized by the following professional associations: the Association of Massage Therapists Australia, the Australian Acupuncture and Chinese Medicine Association, the Australian Aromatic Medicine Association, the Australian Homeopathic Association, the Australian Natural Therapists Association, Australian Traditional Medicine Society, the International Federation of Aromatherapists (Australian Branch), the National Herbalists Association of Australian (Brisbane branch only), the Reflexology Association of Australia, and the Federation of Chinese Medicine and Acupuncture Societies of Australia. With more than 4000 students and some 260 staff and several public clinics which treat nearly 2000 students a week, Sherwood (2005:134), asserts that ACNM is 'probably the largest natural medicine college in the world'.

At any rate, ACNM has been subsumed into an even larger natural medicine education empire, namely the Endeavour Learning Group, and has been renamed the Endeavour College of Natural Health with campuses in Brisbane, Gold Coast, Melbourne, Perth, Sydney, and Adelaide (www.acnm. edu.au, accessed 3/01/2009). The Endeavour Learning Group also includes Fitnation (an organisation that certifies people to become fitness/personal trainers), the College of Natural Beauty, and the Bay of Plenty College of Homeopathy on the North Island of New Zealand. The Box Hill campus of ACNM apparently has been closed down. The Southern Australian Health Education Centre became part of Endeavour College on 5 December 2008 as Endeavour's Adelaide campus. In the past the Centre offered certificate, diploma, and advanced certificate courses in remedial massage, aromatherapy, Traditional Chinese Medicine remedial massage, nutritional medicine, Western herbal medicine, and naturopathy. Endeavour's Sydney campus had operated as the Sydney College of Homeopathic Medicine, a sister school to the Bay of Plenty College of Homeopathy.

The second largest complementary medical school is the Nature Care College of Naturopathic and Traditional Medicine (est. 1973) located in the St. Leonards section of North Sydney and its second only in size to Australian College of Natural Therapies. It reportedly had some 2600 students in 2000 (Martyr, 2002:276) and claimed over 3000 students and 160 lecturers in 2004 (www.alternativemedicinecollegeaustralia.com.au/naturopathy.htm). The Nature Cure College offers advanced diplomas in naturopathy, homeopathy, nutritional medicine, and Western herbal medicine. It had formerly offered various bachelor's degrees, including in naturopathy (natural therapy), homoeopathic medicine, Traditional Chinese Medicine, and complementary medicine (Martyr, 2002:15). A graduate of Nature Care College told me that the school had dropped its bachelor's degree program in order to reduce its administrative efforts. Nature Care college is accredited by the Australasian Association of Ayurveda, the Australian Homoeopathic Association (NSW), ANTA, and various other associations.

The Australasian College of Natural Therapies was founded by Peter and Freida Bielik, the latter who had trained as an osteopath, chiropractor, and naturopath, in 1982 as the Eastern Suburbs College of Natural Therapies in Bondi Junction (*Prospectus – Australasian College of Natural Therapies, 2003*). Its main campus is located the Surrey Hills section of Central Sydney and its Natural Health Care Centre is situated at 20 Glebe Point Road. ACNT offers numerous courses in natural medicine and manual therapies and natural beauty therapy. Its degree programs function in articulation with the University of New England and Charles Sturt University. This institution was the founding member of the Australian Traditional-Medicine Society and is the first natural therapies college to offer training opportunities at the Royal Hospital for Women.

The Laws College of Naturopathy and Chiropractic derived from a discontented group of students at the Southern School of Naturopathy who approached Mrs. Laws about the possibility of forming a separate naturopathic school. According to Canaway,

> Mrs Laws with the help of her husband (deceased) established the Laws College of Naturopathy and Chiropractic in 1971 in their home in Canterbury. The school moved briefly to Riverdale Road, before Mrs Laws purchased the current property on Canterbury Road in Ringwood (Canaway, 2007:49).

Sandi Rogers, who had obtained her credentials through correspondence training at the Queensland Institute of Natural Sciences, established yet another small Melbourne-based naturopathic college called the National College of Traditional Medicine in Sunshine in 1989, which eventually became defunct (Canaway, 2007:53).

Other prominent schools of natural therapy include the South Australian College of Natural and Traditional Medicine (est. 1980), the Perth Academy of Natural Therapies (est. 1988), and Gracegrove College (Martyr, 2002: 274–276). [For a more extensive listing with details on various programs of study, see Appendix 3.] Some Australian complementary medicine or natural therapies colleges have had a long history of long-distance education and a few offer classes entirely in this manner (Harris, 2002). Health Schools Australia specializes in distance learning. Many complementary medicine colleges offer rather limited programs of study in specific therapeutic modalities. For example, the College of Complementary Medicine (www.complementary.com.au), which has branches in Sydney and Melbourne, offers a Diploma and Advanced Diploma in holistic kinesiology.

In their overview of the status of Traditional Chinese Medicine in Australia, Bensoussan and Myers (1996:157) reported the existence of three Chinese medicine programs of study within public universities and ten in private colleges. Table 8 lists those institutions the offer courses in acupuncture or Chinese herbal medicine that entail more than 800 contact hours. Table 9 lists schools that offered courses in acupuncture or Chinese medicine in 1996.

Table 8 Teaching institutions offering courses in acupuncture or Chinese herbal medicine in 1996*

1. Academy of TCM in Australia (VIC), Advanced Diploma of TCM, non-government accredited
2. Academy of Natural Therapies (Burleigh, QLD), Diploma of Applied (Science), government accredited
3. Australian College of Natural Medicine (Brisbane), Diploma of Applied Science, government accredited
4. Australian Institute of Applied Sciences (Stone's Centre, QLD), Diploma of Applied Science (Acupuncture), government accredited
5. College of Traditional Chinese Medicine Australia (VIC), Diploma of TCM, non-government accredited
6. Hepburn's College of Applied Sciences (South Brisbane), Diploma of Applied Science (Traditional Chinese Medicine), government accredited
7. Melbourne College of Natural Medicine, Diploma of Applied Sciences (Acupuncture), government accredited, p. 2
8. RMIT – Bachelor of Applied Science (Human Biology – Chinese Medicine); Bachelor of Applied Science (Chinese Medicine); Master of Applied Science in Clinical Practice (Acupuncture), government accredited
9. Sydney College of TCM, Diploma of TCM, non-government accredited
10. University of Technology, Sydney – Bachelor of Health Sciences (Acupuncture) and Graduate Diploma of Health Sciences (Acupuncture), government accredited
11. Victoria University of Technology – Bachelor of Health Science (TCM – Acupuncture and Chinese herbal medicine) and Graduate Diploma in Clinical Acupuncture, government accredited
12. South Australian College of Natural Therapies and TCM – Diplomas of Applied Science (TCM), Diploma of Applied Science (Acupuncture), and Diploma of Applied Science (Oriental Remedial Therapies), all government accredited

*Adapted from Bensoussan and Myers (1996:158)

Table 9 Public universities with degrees (either bachelors or masters or both) in CM systems in 2009

University	DC	DO	TCM	ND	HM
RMIT University	x	x	x		
Macquarie University	x				
Southern Cross University		x		x	
University of Western Sydney		x	x	x	
University of Technology, Sydney			x		
University of Sydney					x
Victoria University of Technology		x	x		

The Sydney Institute of Traditional Chinese Medicine offers the Bachelor of Applied Science (TCM) or Masters Degree in TCM in partnership with the University of Western Sydney and is registered as an accredited Diploma of Traditional Chinese Medicine by the New South Wales Accreditation

Board (http://users.bigpond.net.au). An increasing number of institutions have been including instruction in Chinese herbal medicine along with acupuncture in their programs of study (Bensoussan & Myers, 1996:159). Most Australian Chinese medicine programs also maintain links with Chinese schools and hospitals (Bensoussan & Myers, 1996:160).

Most private colleges offering courses in naturopathy and Western medicine offer qualifications at the certificate, diploma, and advanced diploma levels, although a few, such as the Southern School of Natural Therapies and the Australian College of Natural Medicine, offer bachelor's degrees in naturopathy (McCabe, 2005b:120).

Public tertiary institutions offering programs in complementary medicine

The Government began formal recognition of natural health schools in 1992. It implemented National Health Training Packages that include standard qualification titles, such as Advanced Diploma of Naturopathy or Advanced Diploma of Western Herbalism. The Australian government has gone further than perhaps any other government in a developed society in supporting public education in complementary, not only chiropractic, osteopathy, and Chinese medicine (in the case of Victoria), but also an array of natural therapies. It has done so in the following four ways: (1) by creating degree programs in various complementary medical systems in public universities; (2) by creating partnerships with private complementary medicine schools that lead to degrees in addition to advanced diplomas; (3) by offering advanced diplomas in various complementary medicines, particularly naturopathy, at TAFEs or public vocational institutions; and (4) by having authorized some private colleges to offer degrees in certain complementary medicine systems.

Table 9 depicts public universities with degree programs in various complementary medicine systems [See Appendix 4 for more details on these programs of study]. Four TAFEs or public vocational schools also offer advanced diplomas in various complementary medical systems, including all of them in naturopathy.

Table 10 depicts various public universities offering partnership extension programs enabling complementary medicine practitioners with advanced diplomas to earn bachelors degrees. Southern Cross University started the first naturopathic training program in an Australian public university in 1997 and the first naturopathic training program in a public university in the world. While various public universities initially enthusiastically embraced complementary medicine programs, some of them have

Table 10 Public universities offering partnership extension programs enabling complementary medicine practitioners with advanced diplomas to earn bachelors degrees in 2009

1. Charles Sturt University (Bachelor of Health Sciences – Complementary Medicine)
2. Southern Cross University (Bachelor of Natural Therapies)
3. University of New England (Bachelor of Health Science in Naturopathy, TCM, or Homeopathic Medicine)
4. Victoria University (Bachelor of Science – Natural Medicine)*
5. University of Newcastle (Bachelor of Natural Therapies)
6. University of Western Sydney (Bachelor of Health Sciences in Naturopathy)

*This program was dropped relatively recently

been terminated for various reasons. In 1997 Victoria University created a Bachelor of Health Science – Natural Medicine – Conversion Course (www.staff.vu.edu.au/natmed/NatMed.htm, access 18/02/2006). Until its closure sometime 2006, the course allowed students with a diploma or advanced diploma in various natural therapies, including massage, acupuncture, naturopathy, homeopathy, myotherapy, hypnosis, and Chinese herbal medicine, to upgrade their credentials to a bachelor's degree and theoretically even a master's or PhD degree. Most classes were held at the St. Albans campus on Tuesday and Thursday from 5:30 to 8:30 pm. Like the naturopathic bachelor's degree program, one reason that this program did not attract more students was its location in an outer western suburb of Melbourne. Elsewhere in Melbourne, La Trobe University operated a combined nursing/naturopathy program in which students took their nursing subjects at the Bundoora campus and their naturopathic subjects at the Southern School of Natural Therapies situated in the inner-city suburb of Fitzroy. This program ceased admitting students a few years ago and the later of its students are presently completing their naturopathic training at SSNT. Finally, the University of Newcastle reportedly terminated a degree program in Western herbal medicine for budgetary reasons.

The School [now a department as opposed to a school] of Natural and Complementary Medicine at Southern Cross University developed a Basic Model of (W)holistic Medicine in 1999. In contrast to a strong tendency within the holistic health movement to engage in a holism that focuses on mind-body-spirit connections, the SCU model asserts that,

> It is also important to recognise that the individual does not exist in isolation. In this model the individual is placed in a social and ecological continuum of family, community and environment. Here family is defined as all the important relationships in an individual's life; community as the broader social group or groups of which the individual is a part; and environment as the physical ecosystem in which the

individual lives. In total six elements of whole-person care have been defined: (1) physical; (2) mental; (3) spiritual; (4) family; (5) community; and (6) environment (Myers, Hunter, Snider, & Zeff., 2003:56).

The naturopathic program at Southern Cross University is unique in being the only one in Australia in which its students obtain clinical experience in a public hospital, namely St. Vincent's Hospital Lismore (Weir, 2005:334).

Publicly funded training programs in complementary medicine appear to pose a financial threat to the private schools of complementary medicine and may be a factor prompting the latter to upgrade their requirements. When Hans Wohlmuth served as the Acting Head of the School of Natural and Complementary Medicine at Southern Cross University, he stated in an interview,

> Although Australia undoubtedly has been at the forefront of natural therapies education for many years, there is no doubt that the quality of training on offer has been highly variable. Again, from the public perspective, there needs to be more uniform educational standards. There is no doubt in mind that the future minimum educational requirement for practitioners such as naturopaths, herbalists and nutritionists will be a bachelor degree. Of course the majority of practitioners do not currently have degree qualifications, but there are ways in which they can upgrade their qualifications and this would require a regulatory requirement sometime in the future. At Southern Cross University, we offer an external degree upgrade programme, the Bachelor of Natural Therapies, which has been specifically designed for qualified natural therapists. The programme recognises previous training and allows practitioners to obtain a degree qualification at their own pace by way of distance education (Courses and colleges. *The Art of Healing – Byron Bay*, Issue 7:28-29).

As the founder of the huge, multi-campus Australian College of Natural Medicine, Peter Sherwood articulates the threat that publicly-funded schools of complementary medicine pose to private institutions,

> In Australia, the natural medicine profession was built by cooperative effort and led by some outstanding individuals. It was entirely the work of the private sector, which faced hostile criticism from the medical establishment, particularly from the universities. Because of the outstanding success of the natural medicine industry, the universities, which receive substantial government subsidies, are now seeking control of natural medicine, education, and, therefore, its professions. Certain government agencies appear to be placing impediments in the path of the private sector, to the advantage of the universities (Sherwood, 2005:334).

He notes that ACNM has spent around $2 million in order to obtain degree accreditation for its programs in naturopathy, Chinese medicine, homeopathy, nutritional medicine, Western herbal medicine, and musculo-skeletal therapy (Sherwood, 2004:226).

The private colleges feel threatened by public universities, such as Charles Sturt University and the University of New England, which allow the graduates of the former to upgrade their credentials to the degree level by taking additional courses, generally online ones. Powell (2003:8), a consultant to the Australian College of Natural Medicine, argues that public universities may eventually drive the private colleges out of the complementary medicine business. McCabe describes the competitive nature of complementary medicine education, at least as it pertains to naturopathy and Western medicine, in the following terms,

> The failure of the profession to unite behind a bachelor's degree as the minimum preparation for practitioners – a movement that began in the 1980s – has led to the present situation whereby the lack of common educational standard contributes to ineffective self-regulation and increases the need for independent external regulation. Educational policy has, to a considerable extent, been influenced by individuals who have a common commercial interest in education and who therefore have a substantial conflict of interest (McCabe, 2005b:151).

At any rate, an increasing number of students are opting to obtain bachelor's degrees rather than advanced diplomas or diplomas in naturopathy and Western herbal medicine as Table 11 below indicates.

Whereas in the past, most naturopaths or Western herbalists obtained either a diploma or advanced diploma, Table 11 indicates that growing trend has been for higher qualifications in complementary medicine training, a

Table 11 Student enrolments in diploma, advanced diploma, bachelor degree, and bachelor degree conversion programs in naturopathy and western herbal medicine (WHM) in 2003*

Course type	Number of campuses	Advanced diplomas enrolments	Bachelor's degree enrolments
Advanced Diploma in Naturopathy	17	1254	
Advanced Diploma in WHM	12	348	
Total Advanced Diploma		1602	
Bachelor's Degree in Naturopathy	7		1372
Bachelor's Degree in WHM	1		40
Total Bachelor's Degree			1412
Bachelor's Degree Conversions	4		553

*Adapted from McCabe (2005b:131)

trend which tends to favour public universities in an increasingly competitive market. Furthermore, two campuses offer graduate certificates master's degrees and three campuses offer PhD degrees in either naturopathy or Western herbal medicine. Despite an emphasis on greater qualifications in naturopathy and Western medicine, many graduates from naturopathic and Western medicine programmes have difficulty translating their education into a viable career. McCabe reports,

> Six education providers provided information on the employment status of graduates. Collection methods for the private colleges were either not stated, or were said to be 'informal' surveys. Two private colleges reported similar figures of 40–50 percent of graduates in either full-time or part-time practice. One added that 'most of the remainder had an intention to practise, others were not intending but were no dissatisfied with that situation'... UNE [University of New England] reported figures collected for 1999–2002, which showed 42–56 percent of graduates in full-time work related to naturopathy or WHM, and 30–38 percent in part-time work related to naturopathy or WHM. SCU [Southern Cross University] provided data from a compulsory higher education survey undertaken twelve months after graduation, which showed that 81 percent were employed and had an average income above $30,000 (McCabe, 2005b:134).

Ironically, despite such sobering data, the Australian College of Natural Medicine, a proprietary institution, in its 2006 course guide made the following claim,

> Career opportunities for graduates are bright because of the worldwide need for qualified practitioners to service the increasing consumer need for natural health care. Graduates of ACNM have proven to be competent, ethical, safe health care professionals and are working throughout Australia and overseas in a range of fields (Australian College of Natural Medicine, 2006:25).

As Table 12 indicates, only a small minority of teaching staff in naturopathic and Western herbal medicine programmes are employed on a full-time basis.

	Type of training institution	Full-time	Part-time	Sessional	Guest
Table 12 Teaching staff in naturopathic and western medicine training programmes*	Private colleges	17 (2.5%)	29 (4%)	531 (74.5%)	134 (19%)
	Universities	16 (19%)	15 (18%)	47 (55%)	7 (8%)
	TAFEs	3 (12%)	10 (42%)	11 (46%)	0

*Adapted from McCabe (2005b:138)

Complementary medicine research occurs at several institutions. The Australian Centre for Complementary Medicine Education and Research (ACCMER) has two sites – the University of Queensland Office at Mater Health Services Building in Brisbane and the New South Wales Office at Southern Cross University in Lismore. It conducts clinical efficacy trials and social research on complementary medicine groups and offers both masters and PhD programs.

The Herbal Medicines Research and Education Centre (est. 1997) based at the University of Sydney conducts efficacy studies on herbal and other complementary medicines and offers a master of Herbal Medicines (www. pharm.ysyd.edu.au/hmrec/program.htm, accessed 30/04/2004. The Centre for Complementary Medicine Research situated at the University of Western Sydney conducts clinical efficacy studies and public health and social health research on complementary medicine (www.uws.edu.au/research/researchcentres/ccmr, accessed 23/02/2004). Between 1999 and 2003, ACCMER received $1,118,859 in research grants, all of it from the private sector (McCabe, 2005b:140).

Summary

This chapter has provided a cursory overview of both private and public institutions offering courses in complementary medicine. The emergence of complementary medicine programs offering bachelor's degrees at public universities appears to have contributed to the upgrading of programs of study at the private schools. This is evidenced by the fact that various private institutions have formed partnerships with public universities, particularly the University of New England and Charles Sturt University, so that their students may obtain the baccalaureate degree. Much research on the nature of education and socialization into the role of complementary practitioner at both private and public institutions as well as the social characteristics of their students is needed. Another issue that needs to be addressed is the tensions that may have developed between the private and public institutions as they seek to attract students to their respective programs and place them into a medical marketplace that may now be glutted with complementary practitioners seeking clients.

Chapter 6

Australian dominative medicine and complementary medical practices

Introduction

In contrast to simple pre-industrial or Indigenous societies, which tend to exhibit a more-or-less coherent medical system, the state or complex societies manifest the coexistence of an array of medical systems or a pattern of *medical pluralism*. From this perspective, *the* medical system of a society consists of the totality medical sub-systems that coexist in a cooperative or competitive relationship with one another. In post-industrial societies, one finds, in addition to biomedicine – as this book has demonstrated in the case of Australia – other systems such as homeopathy, chiropractic, Western herbalism, naturopathy as well as religious and folk healing systems. In keeping with Navarro's (1986:1) assertion that classes as well as races, ethnic groups, and genders within capitalist societies 'have different ideologies which appear in different forms of cultures', it may be argued that these social categories also construct different medical systems which coincide with their respective views of reality. Bearing this thought in mind, medical pluralism tends to exemplify hierarchical relations in the larger society; only ones based on class, caste, racial, ethnic, regional, religious, and gender distinctions. National medical systems in the modern world tend to be *plural* rather than *pluralistic* in that biomedicine has achieved dominance over heterodox and/or religious and folk medical systems.

In this chapter, I present a working model of medical pluralism in Australian society. I argue that whereas the Australian medical system with its various medical sub-systems was relatively pluralistic in the nineteenth century, by the early twentieth century it had evolved into a dominative system in which biomedicine achieved dominance over other medical sub-systems. As noted in Chapter 1, regular medicine or what became biomedicine formed associations of members to challenge competition, lobby the state to ban or at least restrict heterodox practitioners (who were called 'quacks'), built alliances with conservative forces in the government, and monopolize state funding for education and research on health-related issues. Nevertheless, biomedical dominance over rival medical systems in any modern society, including Australia, has never been absolute. The state must periodically make concessions to subordinate social groups in the interest of maintaining social order.

Elsewhere I have argued that the US dominative medical system reflects class, racial, ethnic, and gender relations in the larger society in that the practitioners of more prestigious medical sub-systems, such as biomedicine and osteopathic medicine as a parallel medical system, tend to be white males of higher socio-economic categories, practitioners of folk medical systems tend to be lower-class females of colour (Baer, 2001). In that Australia is an advanced capitalist and multi-ethnic society like the United States, I suspect that much of the same could be said of its dominative medical system, and some of the evidence presented in this chapter indicates that this indeed is the case. Figure 1 below depicts a model of the Australian dominative medicine system.

Figure 1
The Australian dominative medical system

Biomedicine

Fully-legitimised professionalised heterodox medical systems
 Chiropractic
 Osteopathy
 Chinese medicine in Victoria

Semi-legitimised professionalised heterodox medical systems
 Chinese medicine outside of Victoria
 Naturopathy and natural therapies
 Direct-entry midwifery
 Homoeopathy

Limited or marginal heterodox medical systems
 Massage therapy
 Reflexology
 Reiki
 Kinesiology

Religious healing systems
 Spiritualism
 Christian science
 Pentecostalism
 Scientology
 New age healing

Folk and ethnic medical systems
 Anglo-Australian folk medicine
 European immigrant groups' folk medical systems
 Asian folk medical systems
 Aboriginal folk healing systems

The 1996 Census identified some 4,700 complementary practitioners in 1996, 1939 of who were naturopaths, 464 acupuncturists, 259 osteopaths, and 352 'natural therapists' of various sorts (Expert Committee on Complementary Medicines in the Health System, 2003). In contrast, it reported that in 2000, Australia had some 56,000 biomedical physicians, of which about 47,000 were practicing clinicians (Expert Committee, 2003). According to the 2006 Census, there are 8,595 complementary practitioners in Australia, 2,488 of whom are chiropractors, 2,982 naturopaths, 948 acupuncturists, 776 osteopaths, 480 Traditional Chinese Medicine practitioners, and 236 homeopaths (Australian Bureau of Statistics, 2008:2). Not included in these statistics, however, are various other categories of complementary practitioners, such as Western herbalists, direct-entry midwives, massage therapists, and other types of body workers, not to speak of religious and folk healers.

Kevin White (2000) questions the utility of the concept of medical dominance given that the corporatisation of general biomedical practices along with state surveillance procedures have come to greatly curtail the autonomy of biomedical physicians in Australia. Other sociologists have referred to a similar process in the United States as the 'deprofessionalization' or 'proletiarization' of biomedical physicians. These trends have prompted Willis (1988) to speak of a 'modified professional dominance'. While White's observation that biomedicine has undergone a certain decline in authority and power is correct, nevertheless, within the context of the healthcare division of labour, biomedicine continues to exert dominance, in one form or other, over both allied health professionals and complementary practitioners.

Chiropractic and osteopathy as full-legtimised complementary medical systems

Chiropractic and osteopathy constitute fully legitimised heterodox medical systems in that sense that all of their training programs are embedded in public universities and that their practitioners have enjoyed statutory registration since the 1980s in all jurisdictions of Australia. They have been incorporated into the medical division of labour primarily as musculoskeletal specialties. Fazari (1999:55) delineates three camps within Australian chiropractic, namely (1) the 'straights' who focus on spinal adjustment, (2) the 'mixers' who combine spinal adjustment with naturopathic, homeopathic, and other complementary therapies, and (3) the mixers who 'seek to use scientifically proven methods'. Fazari (1999:59) suggests that chiropractors shed their metaphysical concepts and embrace 'their true area of expertise, namely the care of neuromusculoskeletal (meaning musculoskeletal and peripheral nervous system) problems' and view themselves as limited practitioners. While many, if not most, chiropractors in Australia may have indeed followed this course of action to 'gain legitimacy and state patronage, by no means have they backed away from their belief that chiropractice may indeed offer successful treatment for Type O (organic or visceral) disorders [as opposed to Type A (musculoskeletal disorders)] (Eastwood, 1997:85). Chiropractic training programs as well as presumably osteopathic training programs have increasingly become increasingly biomedicalised. For example, a recent comparison of chiropractic and naturopathic training programs in Australia revealed that whereas university naturopathic programs devoted 26.2 percent of their courses to biomedical ones and private naturopathic programs, 23 percent of their courses to biomedical ones, chiropractic programs devoted 45.9 percent of their courses to biomedical ones (Grace, Vemulpad, & Beirman, 2007).

In a similar vein, a perusal of pamphlets and books on osteopathy designed for the general public indicate that it too constitutes a musculoskeletal speciality within the Australian context. In contrast to the osteopaths or osteopath/chiropractors of yesteryear, who incorporated naturopathy into their practices, most Australian osteopaths today by and large emphasise manipulation and soft tissue work in the treatment of back pain and specific conditions such as migraines and asthma (Bowden, 1988; Lucas & Moran, 2003).

This raises the question as to whether chiropractic and osteopathy constitute complementary medical systems or increasingly conventional components of the biomedical division of labour. On the one hand, Ebrall (2003) and Lucas and Moran (2003) have written chapters on chiropractic and osteopathy, respectively, as part of Robson's (2003) anthology on complementary medicine that suggest that they still fall under the large rubric of 'complementary medicine'. Conversely, one might argue that chiropractic and osteopathy have come to resemble dentistry, optometry, podiatry as limited practice professions in terms of scope of practice within the Australia scenario. According to Willis, chiropractic 'achieved politico-legal legitimation in a way which really left medical dominance unchallenged' (Willis, 1989a:191) and 'has been incorporated into health division of labour primarily as a specialist in treatment of one part of the body' (Willis, 1989a:200). Much the same could be said of Australian osteopathy. In describing the status of chiropractic in the United States, Moore (1993:138) argues that it 'has moved into position as the orthodox, non-traditional approach to health – a type of orthodox unorthodoxy' that occupies a niche between biomedicine and the holistic health or the CAM movement. The same argument could be made for both chiropractic and osteopathy in Australia.

Indeed, the earning power of chiropractors and osteopaths suggests that they have achieved a high degree of legitimacy within the context of the Australian dominative medical systems, even if their practices are still regarded as 'unconventional' or 'unorthodox' within some circles, particularly biomedical ones. The Australian Bureau of Statistics (1998:5–7) cited the following statistics for the number and gender composition of the chiropractic and osteopathic professions in Australia for 1997–1998: chiropractors; 1,555 males, 498 females and osteopaths, 284 males, 111 females. O'Neill (1994a:11) describes chiropractic as 'small, well-paid, predominantly male, private practice occupations'. According to the Australian Bureau of Statistics (2008:2), in 2006 32.6 percent of chiropractors were female, whereas 48.7 percent (nearly half) of osteopaths were female. Why osteopathy has become more of a feminised profession rather than chiropractic requires further study.

Chiropractors overwhelmingly claim to have above average annual incomes (Wiesner, 1989:19). Table 13 suggests that chiropractors and osteopaths actually earn higher incomes in Australia than do general biomedical physicians and dentists, despite the fact that they have less formal training.

Duckett notes that '[a]n asterisk (*) indicates that the estimate has a Relative Standard Error (RSE) of greater than 25 percent and care should therefore be exercised in using it' (Duckett, 2004:61). It is increasingly that chiropractors and osteopaths, who are predominantly males, earn considerably more than do physiotherapists, who are predominantly females. His statistics indicate the presence of 2,700* male physiotherapists and 6,600 female physiotherapists. Thus, at least in part, the lower incomes of physiotherapists as opposed to chiropractors and osteopaths may be a result of gender bias.

As for their primary modality, namely, manipulative therapy, O'Neill (1994a:192) observes that it 'has become increasingly popular with other main primary contract practitioners – physiotherapists and registered medical practitioners – who considerably outnumber chiropractors and

Occupation	Mean weekly earnings in main job ($)
General biomedical practitioners	1492
Specialist biomedical practitioners	2517
Registered nurses	713
Dental practitioners	1519
Physiotherapists	704
Chiropractors and osteopaths	1909*

Table 13 Mean weekly earnings in main job for selected health practitioners, 2002

Source: Duckett (2004:61)

osteopaths' (O'Neill, 1994a:12). Chiropractic and osteopathy are reimbursed by various private health insurance plans as well as Medicare on a limited basis and with referral from a biomedical physician.

Despite assertions on part of the chiropractic and osteopathic professions that they are quite distinct entities, the Australian government and the various state and territorial jurisdictions seems to be treating them as co-equals in terms of statutory recognition and funding for training programs. An indication of this policy was the decision of Medicare in 2004 to create new regulations that permit claims by chiropractors and osteopaths, along with physiotherapists and pathologists, on referral of a biomedical practitioner (McCabe, 2005a:29). The Enhanced Primary Care plan permits only five visits per year. As Weir (2005:33) so aptly observes, '[t]he referral requirement for this treatment places control over this provision firmly in the hands of the medical profession'.

Unlike other complementary practitioners, chiropractors and osteopaths may use the title 'Doctor' in all political jurisdictions except Queensland.

Chinese medicine outside of Victoria, naturopathy or natural therapies, and direct-entry midwifery as partially legitimised heterodox medical system

In contrast to chiropractic and osteopathy and Chinese medicine in Victoria, Chinese medicine outside of Victoria, naturopathy or the natural therapies, and direct-entry midwifery constitute semi-legitimised professionalised heterodox medical systems in that, with the exception of Chinese medicine in Victoria, they have not achieved statutory registration in any Australian jurisdiction. Conversely, they have achieved some degree of legitimation in that an increasing number of their training programs are situated either in public universities or in partnerships between private colleges and public universities. Furthermore, the federal government has granted, at least tentatively, acupuncturists and Chinese medicine practitioners, herbalists, and naturopaths belonging to various professional associations with an exemption from the GST for services rendered. The fact that both the federal government and certain state governments have commissioned various inquiries into various aspects of complementary medicine constitutes a de-facto type of legitimation.

Chinese medicine and acupuncture

Acupuncturists and Chinese medicine practitioners find themselves in competition with many other practitioners, including chiropractors, osteopaths, and natural therapists, physiotherapists, biomedical physicians

(O'Neill, 1994a:12–13). In other words, although acupuncture constitutes the primary modality of some practitioners, for many others it is an
adjunct within the context of broader scope of practice. Bensoussan and
Myers (1996) conducted a survey that provided a social profile of AACMA
members. Fifty-five percent were male and 45 percent female. In terms of
their first TCM qualification, 60 percent had obtained it in Australia and 40
percent overseas; 30 percent of the respondents were of ethnic Chinese
background.

    Bensoussan and Myers (1996) also conducted a survey based on a mail-
ing list generated in from associations representing Chinese medicine practitioners. Out of 2,075 names on the list, 1,074 practitioners responded to
survey. As many as 433 (40 percent) designated TCM as their primary health
practice; 571 (53 percent) designated their main health practice in another
discipline. The respondents included 426 biomedical physicians. Other
practitioners who practiced acupuncture in the sample included physiotherapists, chiropractors, naturopaths, nurses, massage therapists, medical
specialists, osteopaths, etc. Males accounted for 63 percent of the primary
Chinese medicine practitioners and 73 percent of the non-primary Chinese
medicine workforce. Table 14 depicts specifics of the work profiles of the
respondents.

    The Australian Bureau Statistics (2008:643) reported that in 2006, 49.5
percent of acupuncturists were female, whereas 41.7 percent of Traditional
Chinese Medicine practitioners were female.

Occupation	Number	Percent of workforce
Primary TCM practitioners	433	40.3
Non-primary TCM practitioners	571	53.2
General practitioners	411	38.3
Physiotherapist	29	2.7
Chiropractor	24	2.2
Nurse	21	2.2
Medical specialist	15	1.4
Massage therapist	14	1.3
Osteopath	6	0.6
Homeopath	4	0.4
Counsellor/psychologist	2	0.2
Western herbalist	1	0.1
Other	16	1.5
Missing or other than one occupation	70	6.5
Total	1074	100.0

Table 14 Work profiles of TCM practitioners: primary and non-primary*

*Bensoussan and Myers (1996:3–8)

Alan Bensoussan is one of the foremost TCM practitioners in Australia. He earned his undergraduate degree in physics and applied mathematics (Bennett, 2002–2003:33). Afterward he did three years of acupuncture study in Sydney in early 1980s and authored the first Australian text in English on acupuncture research methodology (A Member profile. *Newsletter of the Australian and Chinese Medicine Association Ltd*, June 2004, pp. 10–11). Bensoussan (1989) published *The Vital Meridian* and is the principal author of *Towards a Safer Choice: The Practice of Traditional Chinese Medicine in Australia*, the workforce study that led to registration of TCM in Victoria. He presently is an Associate Professor at the University of Western Sydney, the Head of the UWS Chinese Medicine Unit, and Director of CompleMED, a UWS research centre.

Naturopathy or the natural therapies

The Social Development Committee commissioned by the Parliament of Victoria provided an early survey of natural therapists in Victoria. It drew its sample of 278 practitioners from the membership lists of the ANTA, the ATMS, the Acupuncture Ethics and Standards Organisation, the Australian Homeopathic Association, the Australian Naturopathic Practitioners and Chiropractors Association, and the Homeopathic Society of Australia; entries in the Yellow Pages telephone directory under the headings of naturopath, herbalist, homeopath, and acupuncturist, and a list of recent graduates of the Southern School of Natural Therapies (Social Development and Committee, 1986:80). Fifty-six percent (155) of the respondents described themselves as naturopaths, 19 percent (53) as acupuncturists, 17 percent (48) as homeopaths, 14 percent (39) as naturopaths, 9 percent (26) as chiropractors, and small percentages as practitioners of other natural therapies; some respondents identified themselves with multiple labels (Social Development Committee, 1986:80–81). Forty percent of the respondents, more so in the case of women, claimed that they practiced complementary medicine on a part-time basis (Social Development Committee, 1986:82).

Sociologist Diane Wiesner (1981:38) presents the following portray of the old-time Australian naturopath or natural therapist in Australia: 'The typical naturopathic practitioner is male, is drawn from a middle to upper socio-economic and educational strata of society and enjoys a ranking in the status hierarchy which is on a par with other health-related personnel such as physiotherapists, but below that of medical doctors and graduates of acknowledge tertiary institutions, such as pharmacists and nurses'. The old-time naturopaths generally either owned their own clinics or worked in partnerships with chiropractors or acupuncturists, tended to be self-trained or supplemented their interests in various therapeutic modalities, such as dietetics and iridology, 'with part-time diplomas obtained in Australia or from the USA' (Wiesner, 1981:38).

By the 1970s, a younger generation of naturopaths had emerged with training from an assortment of naturopathic or natural therapy colleges. The Director of Education at what was then the College of Osteopathic and Natural Therapies in the St. Leonards suburb of Sydney reported 'that presently enrolled students were considerably younger than in previous years, were often choosing to undergo training in natural therapy with a view to making it a career and were not necessarily committed to or initially convinced of, the beliefs and the benefits' (Wiesner, 1981:39).

Furthermore, whereas in its early days Australian naturopathy was largely a male-dominated occupation, it has evolved into a predominantly female endeavour. Alf Jacka, a prominent naturopath, made the following observation about the naturopathic education scene in the 1970s and early 1980s,

> During the last ten years particularly, the ratio of females to males has changed greatly; so much that currently the Southern School of Natural Therapies there are many more female students than males. For example, in the present second year class the ratio is four to one (Jacka, 1983:3).

My visits to the School of Natural and Complementary Medicine at Southern Cross University, the Southern School of Natural Therapies, and the Melbourne branch of the Australian College of Natural Medicine indicate that the situation some two decades later has not changed appreciably. The Australian Bureau of Statistics (2008:2) reports that in 2006, 79.0 percent of naturopaths were female.

Two major surveys of naturopaths and other natural therapists have been conducted in Australia. The first one headed by Ann Hale (2002) entailed a survey conducted in collaboration with the Australian Traditional Medicine Society. It was sent to 1,500 members of the Australian Natural Therapists Association, with 713 of them responding. Of these, those respondents who were not accredited in naturopathy, herbal medicine, acupuncture, or Traditional Chinese Medicine were excluded, resulting in a final sample of 614, 69.5 percent of who were women. The primary discipline accreditations in rank order were naturopathy (76.4 percent), naturopathy and Western herbal medicine (10.6 percent), acupuncture and TCM (6.4 percent), and Western herbal medicine (2.1 percent). 38.6 percent of the ANTA members held membership in another complementary medicine association. For example, 91 (14.8 percent) members belonged to the National Herbalists

Association of Australia. As many as 90.7 percent of the same were practicing and 9.3 percent were not (Hale, 2002:17). Table 15 depicts the number of consultations conducted by practitioners in an average week and Table 16 depicts the academic qualifications of the respondents.

There appears to be an upgrading process going on in terms of academic qualifications expected of natural therapists, with public universities driving this process prompting some private colleges to follow suit.

Bensoussan et al. (2004) conducted a workforce survey naturopaths and Western herbalists in Australia. They mailed 3,540 survey forms to practitioners on the list of the Grand United Health Fund, which is one of first insurers to provide benefits to members for complementary medicine services; 423 surveys were returned. Of the remaining 3,117 surveys, 795 were completed. Table 17 indicates that many respondents referred to themselves by more than one practitioner designation.

Table 15
Number of consultations by practitioners in an average week*

	Frequency	Percent	Cumulative Percent
1–5	97	17.5	17.5
6–10	89	16.1	33.6
11–20	122	22.0	55.6
21–30	100	18.1	73.6
31–40	67	12.1	85.7
40+	79	14.3	100.0
Total	554	100.0	
No response	27		
Total	581		

*Adapted from Hale (2002:27)

Table 16
Academic qualifications*

Qualification	Number	Percent
Diploma	317	51.8
Advanced diploma	115	18.8
Bachelor in some complementary therapy	105	17.2
Qualification in acupuncture and naturopathy or herbalism	17	2.8
Overseas diploma	17	2.8
Grandfather provision	13	2.1
Overseas degree	12	2.0
Masters degree	6	1.0
Diploma with bachelor degree in progress	5	0.8
Postgraduate or graduate diploma from tertiary institution	3	0.5
Bachelor and masters degrees	2	0.3

*Adapted from Hale (2002:34)

Title	Number	Percent
Herbalist	489	61.5
Naturopath	604	76.0
Homeopath	208	26.2
Nutritionist	315	39.6
Massage therapist	277	34.8
Bach flowers practitioner	175	22.0

*Adapted from Bensoussan et al. (2004)

Income $	Number	Percent
<20,000	172	21.6
20,001–40,000	137	17.2
40,001–60,000	218	27.4
60,001–80,000	72	9.1
80,001–100,000	55	6.9
100,000+	30	3.8

*Adapted from Bensoussan et al. (2004:22)

Percentage	Number	Percent
<20	129	16.2
21–40	99	12.5
41–60	114	14.3
61–80	106	13.3
81–100	323	40.6

*Adapted from Bensoussan et al. (2004:22)

In addition to those designations listed in Table 17, respondents listed various other designations, including aromatherapist, meditation/relaxation specialist, medical specialist, general medical practitioner, pharmacist, chiropractor, osteopath, physiotherapist, nurse, counsellor, psychologist, and Traditional Chinese Medicine practitioner.

Tables 18 and 19 delineate income earnings and percent of gross income from naturopathic and Western herbal practices in Australia.

Over fifteen years ago, Wiesner (1989:19) reported that naturopaths, homeopaths, and herbalist are 'generally barely able to make living'. While this assertion may not be quite as true today, the evidence in Tables 16 and 17 suggest that many natural therapists continue to struggle to make a decent income and that many are forced to supplement the incomes from their practices with other forms of income. For example, Ondine Spitzer (2002), an herbalist and naturopath, practiced in a complementary health centre in Moonee Ponds, Victoria, and lectured in herbal medicine and supervised a student clinic at the Australian of Natural Medicine. She also served as the President of the Victorian Herbalists Association and earned an MA in Social Health (Medical Anthropology) at the University of Melbourne (personal communication). Gill Stannard (2002:1) works as a naturopath in City Natural Therapies – a group practice in central Melbourne that includes another naturopath, a massage therapist, and two osteopaths.

It should be noted that natural therapeutics is filled with numerous 'success stories', not merely in monetary terms but also in terms of contributions to the profession. Judy Jacka (1998) authored *Natural Therapies – The Politics and the Passion*, an account that blends her personal journey in naturopathy with the politics of the Southern School of Natural Therapies and the natural therapies profession in Australia. In the course of investigating Theosophy and other metaphysical systems and spiritual healing, she learned about Alf Jacka, an East Melbourne naturopath, who she visited for a medical check-up. Utilizing iris diagnosis, he informed her that her lymphatic system was congested and nervous system depleted and prescribed a herbal mixture and a bottle of drops for her, resulting in improvement of her condition (Jacka, 1998:5). While rearing her children, Jacka read books on natural therapeutics on her own for several years before finally deciding to study at Alf's college entitled the Victorian Branch College of the National Association of Naturopaths, Osteopaths, and Chiropractors (Jacka, 1998:10–13). Following graduation from the college in 1971, Jacka developed a successful practice in the Kew section of Melbourne in which by her fifth year she was treating some ninety patients a week (Jacka, 1998:20). During this time she divorced her husband and married her physician and mentor Alf Jacka and took over the operation of the association college and renamed it the Southern School of Naturopathy (Jacka, 1998:22). Judy Jacka served as director of the college and also taught various courses at the college while Alf continued on as the Dean. She was one of the 93 individuals interviewed by the Webb Committee and also published various books on naturopathic philosophy and natural therapies including *Frontiers of Natural Therapies: A Bridge between Ancient Wisdom and New Edges of Science* (1989). She also served as a consultant in the creation of the first naturopathic training program at a public Australian university, namely the School of Natural and Complementary Medicine at Southern Cross University (Jacka, 1998:163).

Based on an interviews with Assunta Hunter, a well-known Australian naturopath and naturopathic educator, Canaway (2007:30) suggests that the 'reasons people become naturopaths are possibly changing'. Whereas in the past individuals may have chosen to become naturopaths for political or lifestyle reasons, many naturopathic students view themselves as pursuing a career path, one that even has a certain scientific respectability. Nevertheless, another informant indicated that others who choose to become natural therapists escape the 'corporate witch-hunt mentality that they've been caught up in' (quoted in Canaway, 2007:30). Obviously more research on the social forces that propel individuals to pursue careers in naturopathy and other complementary medical systems is needed.

While the natural therapies and complementary medicine is filled with people struggling to make a living at their chosen career, there are numerous 'success stories'. For example, Stephen Myers, who studied naturopathy and later earned a PhD in Pharmacology and a biomedical degree, served as the principal founder of the School of Natural and Complementary Medicine at Southern Cross University. He worked in the environmental movement in his late teens and early 20s and helped to establish Friends of the Earth Australia in 1974 (Bennett, 2003–2004:13). In 1978, at age 24 he enrolled at the Southern School of Natural Therapies in Melbourne. After graduating at age 28, Myers entered naturopathic practice and formulated products for Blackmores (Bennett, 2003–2004:14). He also studied biomedicine at the University of Newcastle and worked for three years running the night casualty unit at Tamworth Base Hospital.

Myers, along with Alan Bensoussan, co-authored *Towards a Safer Choice*, a review of Chinese medicine in the Australia for the Victorian, New South Wales, and Queensland governments (Bensoussan & Myers, 1996). This document helped to pave the way for the statutory registration of Chinese medicine practitioners and acupuncturists in Victoria in 2000. After helping to develop the curriculum for the Bachelor of Naturopathy Degree at Southern Cross University, he became the Founding Head of School in 1997 (Bennett, 2003–2004:15). Myers has been serving for several years as the Foundation Director of the Australian Centre for Complementary Medicine Education and Research (ACCME) – a joint program between the University of Queensland and Southern Cross Years. In 1997, he was appointed to the Commonwealth Government's Expert Committee on Complementary Medicine in the Health System, an advisory board to the Therapeutic Goods Administration. Myers (2006) has been a vocal advocate of integrative medicine – an approach that seeks to blend together the best of biomedicine and complementary medicine and which is discussed in greater detail later in this book.

Sue Evans (2000a), a lecturer in the School of Natural and Complementary Medicine at Southern Cross University, studied sociology as an undergraduate student, underwent training in herbal medicine in England in the late

1970s, practised in one of first integrative medical clinics in Australia, taught herbal medicine at the Southern School of Natural Therapies in Melbourne, and serves on the board of the National Herbalists Association of Australia. She has essentially blended careers as a practitioner and teacher in both Western herbalism and naturopathy.

Carol Langley established the Allcare Naturopathic Centre in Bexley North (inner southwest Sydney)(Khoury, 2001b:113). She had studied naturopathy from 1986 to 1990 at the South Australian College of Natural Therapies and Traditional Chinese Medicine in Adelaide. In 2001, Langley charged $55 for an initial one-hour visit, $40 for follow-up half-hour visits, $52 for follow-up hour visits, and $60 for 1.5 hour follow-up visits (Khoury, 2001b:114). She usually gave remedial therapy, either massage, reflexology, or auriculotheray, with all follow-up consultations. Her practice focuses on herbal medicine, iridology, massage, and reflexology, but she also used nutrition, homeopathy, aromatherapy, Bowen and Bach flower remedies.

Despite these success stories, there is reason to believe that the complementary medicine marketplace is being glutted, given the large numbers of programs of complementary medicine being offered in both public and private institutions. Indeed, several natural therapists have indicated that this indeed the case in my conversations with them. Although further research is warranted, there is reason to believe that the Australian scenario parallels the dilemma faced by 'complementary and alternative' practitioner in the UK where, according to Stone and Heller (2005:372), '[a]s new training courses are developed for potential CAM practitioners, the therapists of the future are entering a competitive market where earnings may not be as high as the students imagined'.

Lay or direct-entry (non-nursing) midwifery

Although there are a large number of nurse-midwives in Australia, as in other Western societies, the women's liberation movement stimulated development of the natural childbirth movement in Australia. Organisations that grew out of this development included the Childbirth Education Association, the Parents Centres Australia, and The Nursing Mothers Association of Australia (Sutton, 2004:4–5). Several universities, such as Flinders University in Adelaide and Monash University in Melbourne, came to offer direct-entry programs in which midwifery is offered as an undergraduate degree (Sutton, 2004:6). Organisations that promoted midwifery care in both in hospital and home environment include the Australian College of Midwives, the Australian Society of Independent Midwives, a consumer group called Maternity Coalition, and the Community Midwifery Program which since 1990 has been funded by Government to seek alternative models of childbirth for low-risk women (Sutton, 2004:6–7).

Limited or marginal heterodox, religious, and folk medical systems

While some information exists on the social profiles of osteopaths, chiropractors, Chinese Medicine practitioners in Australia, naturopaths, and certain natural therapists, very little exists on various other complementary practitioners, such as homeopaths, body workers, reflexologists, Ayurvedic medicine practitioners, religious healers, and folk healers.

Despite the fact that homeopaths have not developed strong professional associations, they have achieved some legitimacy in Australia. The Australian Homeopathic Association was established in 1995 but evolved from the merger of various earlier homeopathic associations dating back to 1946 (www.homoeopathyoz.org, accessed 3/01/2009). Its sixth conference occurred in Sydney on 12–14 September 2008 in Sydney and featured Peter Fisher, a rheumatologist at the Royal London Homoeopathic Hospital in London. The Australian Bureau of Statistics (2008:2) reports that in 2006, 75.8 percent of homeopaths were female.

The Australian College of Natural Medicine offers a Bachelor of Health Science (Homeopathy) and the University of New England, in partnerships with various private colleges, offers a Bachelor of Health Science (Homeopathic Medicine). Furthermore, various TAFE colleges and numerous private colleges offer qualifications ranging from certificates to advanced diplomas in homeopathy (Weir, 2005:338). Homeopathy is generally included within the training programs in naturopathy or the natural therapies, thus making its status as a distinct primary health endeavour somewhat problematic.

In contrast, massage therapy, Alexander technique, reflexology, aromatherapy, Reiki, polarity therapy, kinesiology, and various other complementary therapies constitute limited or marginal heterodox medical systems for various reasons. Many of these therapeutic systems have become specific treatment modalities that are taught in schools of natural therapy or utilised as adjuncts by natural therapists in their practices. Furthermore, when these systems are taught within the context of a school of natural therapy as a specialised program of study or at a training institution that focuses on a specific therapy, such as aromatherapy or reflexology, they often entail a shorter period of study and the granting of a diploma or certificate rather than a degree or advanced diploma.

Religion	1996	2001
Christian Science	1,494	1,666
Liberal Catholic Church	596	498
Religious Science	634	417
Scientology	1,488	2,032
Spiritualism	8,140	9,279
Theosophy	1,423	1,627

*Adapted Lewis (2005:246)

A paucity of studies exist on various European Australian religious heal-ing systems, such as Christian Science, Spiritualism, Seventh Day Adventism, Pentecostalism, the Liberal Catholic Church, Scientology, New Age healing, and other spiritual healing systems. Christian Science diffused to Australia from the US and reportedly 'by 1910, there were 29 accredited practitio-ners/healers, of whom two-thirds were women' (Sherwood, 2005:133). A New Age online directory of churches and groups lists some 62 Spiritualist churches, spiritual healing groups, and spiritual centres in Australia (Martyr, 2002:306). Fortunately, the Australian census, unlike the US census, includes statistics on new religions. Table 20 depicts membership figures for various Australian religious healing sects in 1996 and 2001.

According to sociologist Gary Bouma, the rise of two primarily European Australian religious healing systems, namely,

> Pentecostal Christianity and New Age religious groups provide the strongest evidence of the impact of [a] major cultural change on Australia's religious and spiritual life... Pentecostal Christianity and many of the New Age religious groups are religions of self-help, offer-ing success theologies, focused on wholeness for the person and requir-ing emotional honesty rather than intellectual rigour – celebration, not cerebration (Bouma, 2006:92).

Pentecostal and other evangelical mega-churches, such as Hillsong in Sydney and the Church of Exurbent Life, have increasingly become com-monplace in Australian capital cities (Bouma, 2006:149–154).

As indicated earlier, religious healers, such as Spiritualists, Christian Science practitioners, and New Age healers, tend to be female. Folk healers in both Indigenous and state societies are often women and presumably this is the case in Australia, but there still exists very little data on this matter. Although I have dealt with religious and folk healing systems only in pass-ing in this book, it is important to stress that they constitute complemen-tary medical systems to which a substantial number of Australians turn in addressing health concerns.

Summary

Medical pluralism in Australia evolved from a relatively pluralistic system in the nineteenth century into a plural or dominative system in the twentieth century and continuing into the twenty-first century. In some ways, the Australian dominative medical system reflects class, racial, ethnic, and gender divisions in the larger society, both in terms of practitioners and patients who access complementary systems. In terms of practitioners, chiropractic and osteopathy still constitute males preserves with Chinese medicine being roughly 50/50 in terms of gender balance. Conversely, most naturopaths, Western herbalists, homeopaths, body workers, energy healers, and religious healers are women.

Chapter 7

Mainstreaming complementary medicine in Australia

Introduction

Although alternative medical systems and therapies have existed on the margins of mainstream society, upper and upper-middle class people with disposable incomes have turned to them since the 1970s. Thus, biomedical physicians, nurses, biomedical and nursing schools, private health insurance companies, and pharmaceutical companies – in part driven by the economic imperative inherent in capitalist societies, and sometimes driven by a paradigm shift in health care that recognises that biomedicine manifests limitations in the treatment of certain disorders, such as cancer and a wide range of chronic diseases – have come to express an increasing interest in them. Willis (1989b:266–270) argues that a process of convergence has emerged between biomedicine and complementary medicine under which four sub-processes have occurred: (1) a growing tendency on the part of complementary practitioners to utilise certain biomedical procedures, such as taking patient histories, blood pressure readings, and conducting physical examinations; (2) a greater recognition of the limitations of a specific complementary modality by referring a patient to a biomedical physician; (3) the adoption of complementary modalities by some biomedical physicians; and (4) a growing de-emphasis on how theoretically compatible (or 'commensurable') or incompatible ('incommensurable') biomedical and complementary modalities are. He argues that 'clinical legitimacy has become increasingly important as the basis of politico-legal legitimation, and has come to assume greater importance than scientific legitimacy, thus making the overall issue of the extent of incommensurability less central in assessing politico-legal legitimacy' (Willis, 1989b:269).

The interest of biomedicine and nursing in complementary medicine

In the past the Australian Medical Association (AMA) had been a virulent opponent of complementary medicine. In 1992, the President of the AMA stated in an SBS television program that '[t]there's no real indication that they [complementary practitioners] are doing anything for people… There's a lot of dishonesty in the alternative medicine area' (quoted in Easthope, 2004:332). In 1992, the AMA published *Chiropractic in Australia* in which it stated

> that a medical practitioner should at all times practise methods of treatment based on sound scientific principles, and accordingly does not recognise any exclusive dogma such as homeopathy, osteopathy, chiropractic or naturopathy (Australian Medical Association, 1992:3).

While the AMA recognised that chiropractors might provide patients with some relief from back pain, it argued 'that chiropractors' use of manipulation to treat pain in the musculoskeletal system involves no more than the application of techniques well known to the medical and physiotherapy professions' (Australian Medical Association, 1992:8). The AMA condemned the chiropractic use of certain forceful manipulative techniques and chiropractic claims in the detection of 'abnormalities in x-rays of spines where these are not apparent to specialist radiologists' (Australian Medical Association, 1992:8). It argued that chiropractic should not qualify for public and private health insurance funding (Australian Medical Association, 1992:9). In addition to its concerted attack upon chiropractic, the AMA had proposed the use of new accreditation rules to refuse Medicare rebates to users of complementary practitioners (Easthope, 1993:289).

Despite the policies of the AMA, many biomedical practitioners have been adopting complementary therapies, especially acupuncture, or are now willing to refer patients to complementary therapists (Easthope, 1993; Easthope, Tranter, & Gill, 2000a). Based upon secondary analysis of 1996 Health Insurance Commission data on clams by GPs for Medicare Benefits Schedule items, Easthope, Beilby, Gill, and Tranter (1998) found that 15.1 percent of them had claimed for acupuncture. In surveys of general practitioners in Victoria and Tasmania, Easthope et al. (2000a) found that in Tasmania 66 percent of general practitioners referred patients to other biomedical physicians, primarily for acupuncture and hypnotherapy, and 55 percent of them referred patients to complementary practitioners, primarily for chiropractic, massage, and osteopathy. In Victoria the referral rate was 93 percent.

Bensoussan and Myers (1996) identify ten programs of study that offer acupuncture training to graduates of biomedical health professions. The Australian Medical Acupuncture Society, Monash University, the Australian Medical Acupuncture College in Sydney, the Royal North Shore Hospital in Sydney, and the Royal Australian College of General Practitioners (Sydney and Melbourne) offer acupuncture courses for biomedical physicians. The

Acupuncture Academy of Western Australia, the Royal Melbourne Institute of Technology, and Edith Cowan University in Perth; the Acupuncture College of Melbourne offer acupuncture courses for health professionals; and the Australian Physiotherapist Association offers course for physiotherapists (Bensoussan & Myers, 1996). The Australian Medical Acupuncture College (est. 1973) has branches in all states and claims a membership of over 750 biomedical physicians (www.acupunctureaustralia.org, accessed 10/11/2008). It publishes the *Journal of the Australian Acupuncture Society.*

In contrast to the US and UK where many biomedical schools offers familiarisation courses on complementary and alternative medicine, Australian biomedical schools have moved slowly in this direction (Owen & Lewith, 2004). The Australian Medical Council has not recommended the teaching of a complementary medicine familiarisation course in biomedical schools. Nevertheless, as Brooks reports,

> Some Australian medical schools are in the process of revising their curricula, with several considering the addition of a CAM component. CAM may be taught as an independent elective, within another unit such as 'society, health and health psychology', or in the teaching of ethics (Brooks, 2004:275).

Discussion of complementary medicine reportedly has been introduced into the undergraduate curriculum of the medical schools at Flinders, Newcastle, Monash, Western Australia and Melbourne universities (Eastwood, 1997:20).

Ironically, as a result of the increasing popularity of complementary medicine, the Australian Medical Association has in recent years relaxed its historical critique of a wide variety of complementary medical systems. Kerryn Phelps, the AMA President, gave a speech at the Healthcare Summit of the Complementary Healthcare Council of Australia in Canberra on 1 March 2001 in which she made the following comments,

> 'One of the conclusions the AMA would like to see come out of a summit like this, is a better relationship between so-called orthodox medicine and so-called alternative or complementary medicine', p. 49.

> 'The AMA and the medical profession has a growing interest in the vast range of alternative and complementary therapies that we believe can help patients and people in our community', p. 49.

> 'But nothing can be achieved through continuing the past adversarial approach between the orthodox and complementary advocates. It's a time I believe to build bridges', p. 49.

'The key to acceptance of complementary medicines as therapies is having an evidence base', p. 49.

'Why the change in policy?... Could the AMA be compromising its staunch adherence to scientific legitimacy in response to consumer demand? With 60% of the population primarily self-prescribing complementary medicines, the interest of consumers is self-evident. Is the AMA's motive to incorporate the practice of complementary medicine, and utilise its medicines, nothing more than economically driven to merely satisfy consumer demand?', p. 52.

In order to foster a dialogue between biomedicine and complementary medicine, Phelps formed the AMA Advisory Committee on Complementary Medicine in 2001.

In 2002, the AMA formally stated that the 'evidence-based aspects of complementary medicine are part of the repertoire of patient care and may have a role in mainstream medical practice', and that 'medical practitioners should be sufficiently well informed about complementary medicine to be able to provide advice to patients.' (Australian Medical Association, 2002). It also called for 'greater regulatory enforcement over the importation and use of raw herbs' and 'appropriate regulation of complementary therapists. Such regulation should ensure that non-medical complementary therapists cannot claim expertise in medical diagnosis and treatment'. The AMA also asserted that biomedical physicians should undergo education about complementary medicine in both their undergraduate studies and through continuing education (Australian Medical Association, 2002:4).

In her address to the International Holistic Health Conference in May 2003, Kerryn Phelps (2003:2), who in her capacity as the President of the AMA from the AMA Complementary Committee, told the audience that she sees a 'place for complementary medicine to work alongside and within orthodox medicine to provide better health outcomes for Australians'. but warned that the Pan scandal dictates that complementary medicine conform to evidence-based standards. Conversely, the Australian Medical Council – the accrediting body for biomedical schools in Australia and New Zealand – adopted a more cautious stance toward complementary therapies in 2000 by referring to them as 'unorthodox', unless they are proven to be efficacious through evidence-based medicine, which automatically makes them 'orthodox by definition, even if the scientific basis of their efficacy is not understood' (quoted in Brooks, 2004:275).

Many biomedical physicians in Australia now offer complementary therapies, particularly acupuncture, spinal manipulation, hypnosis, vitamin therapy, herbal medicine, and homeopathy (Easthope et al., 1998).

Easthope et al. (1998) reports that approximately one-sixth of Australian general practitioners utilise some form of complementary medicine. Based on a questionnaire administered to 290 general practitioners (out of 467 GPs contacted), Easthope et al. (2000a) found that,

> [T]hese results suggest that doctors with favourable attitudes to complementary therapies are more likely to be young and to value holistic approaches in medicine while perceiving complementary therapies to be advantageous in that patients endorse them, they are drug free and have a good palliative rates. Doctors with less favourable attitudes to complementary therapies tend to be older, sceptical of the cure rate claimed for complementary therapies and perceive complementary therapies as having harmful side effects (Easthope, 2000a:1559).

A survey of general practitioners in Perth indicated that the majority felt favourable toward complementary medicine (Hall & Giles-Corti, 2000). In a survey of 488 general practitioners, Pirotta, Cohen, Kotsirilos, and Farish (2000) found that over 80 percent have referred patients to practitioners of acupuncture, hypnosis, and meditation and nearly half have considered applying these therapies to their patients.

As part of a larger study, sociologist Heather Eastwood (1997, 2000) interviewed 17 biomedical general practitioners who utilise complementary therapies. Nine of her respondents 'noted that the consumer demand for alternative medicine had resulted in growing competition from alternative practitioners and/or that doctors were employing alternative medicine to maintain a competitive edge in the face of an oversupply of doctors' (Eastwood, 2000:141). Four GPs 'noted that the oversupply of doctors influenced GP use of alternative medicine. One of the doctors … admitted to offering acupuncture purely as a 'gimmick' to attract patients and to overcome the oversupply of doctors in the market' (Eastwood, 2000:141). Thirteen GPs observed that the consumer demand for complementary medicine is due to increasing preference for natural medicine products rather than synthetic drugs. All of the GPs interviewed 'expressed dissatisfaction and frustration with the adequacy of their biomedical training to equip them to deal with some of their most commonly treated clinical problems' (Eastwood, 2000:143). Three GPS admitted that they treat complementary therapies as adjuncts rather than primary treatment modalities because they tend to be time-consuming. Conversely, eleven of the GPs ignore the 'financial incentive of brief doctor and patient consultation' in opting to utilise complementary therapies in order to provide their patients with the most beneficial treatment (Eastwood, 2000:144). Eastwood's qualitative study indicates that both economic competition from complementary practitioners and a paradigm shift concerning health care were motivating many of her subjects to incorporate complementary therapies in their respective practices. Elsewhere, Eastwood (2004:323) argues that '[m]arket competition, particularly in urban areas of Australia, had led doctors to sign up with general practice commercial providers and also it is, one suspects, although there is not empirical study of this, one of the reasons for incorporating CAM into general practice'.

Bombardieri and Easthope (2000) conducted a survey of the seventy general practices listed in the (Tasmanian) Southern Division of General Practice. Sixty-five of the of practices (93 percent response rate) agreed to participate in the survey (Bombardieri & Easthope, 2000:485). The authors also interviewed thirteen complementary practitioners listed in *Tasmania's Natural Therapy Directory* and the yellow pages. They found that 25 (39 percent) of the general practices offered some kind of complementary therapy and that 33 (19 percent) of the 176 GPs in these practices practised at least one form of complementary therapy; acupuncture was the most commonly used complementary therapy used by 27 GPs (14.5 percent) in twenty (31 percent) of the practices. Bombardieri and Easthope (2000:488) argue that the Hobart results suggest that a weak form of convergence is occurring between biomedicine and complementary medicine in Australia.

More recently, Cohen, Penman, Pirotta, and Da Costa (2005:999) conducted a national survey of 636 Australian general practitioners in which they found that 21 percent reported using various complementary therapies, particularly acupuncture or electroacupuncture, laser, and ultrasound in their practices. They assert that '[n]onmedical therapies, such as acupuncture, massage, meditation, yoga, hypnosis, and chiropractic, are widely used in Australian general practice (Cohen et al., 2005:1003). In terms of various therapies being 'moderately or highly' potentially effective, their respondents gave the following percentages for various therapies: acupuncture 84 percent, aromatherapy 15 percent, Chinese herbal medicine 50 percent, chiropractic 72 percent, herbal medicine 36 percent, homeopathy 18 percent, hypnosis 65 percent, massage 84 percent, meditation 82 percent, naturopathy 29 percent, osteopathy 44 percent, reflexology 10 percent, spiritual healing 19 percent, vitamin and mineral therapy 30 percent, and yoga 76 percent (Cohen et al., 2005:997).

The Australian Complementary Medical Association (ACMA) appears to have been the first formal body of biomedical general practitioners to have been created in Australia. It seeks,

> to join all medical practitioners using preventative, holistic and complementary therapies together in a supported and supportive group to undertake an active role in education of the community and policy

matters regarding the value of complementary medicine in the mainte-
nance of good health and of its valuable position in Australia's medical
system (Easthope et al., 1998).

The absence of a website for this organisation indicates that it may have
become defunct. In the meantime, various biomedical physicians have increasingly come to speak of integrative medicine rather than complementary
and alternative medicine or simply complementary medicine. Like in other
developed societies, more and more biomedical practitioners interested in
complementary therapies speak of 'integrative medicine' – an approach that
supposedly blends together the best features of biomedicine and complementary medicine. In 1992, various biomedical physicians formed the Australian
Integrative Medicine Association that in turn resulted in the Integrative
Medicine Conference in October 1998 (Ngu, 1998). AIMA became the
Australasian Integrative Medicine Association. While its regular members
are biomedical physicians, AIMA allows allied health professionals, such as
physiotherapists, nurses, dieticians, pharmacists and other health workers, to
belong as associate members. The AIMA shares a joint working group with the
Royal Australian College of General Practitioners and has eight special interest groups, including ones in nutritional and environmental medicine, herbal
medicine, and homeopathy (Ngu, 1998:26). Indeed, RACGP began to offer
a course in musculoskeletal medicine and a Certificate in Manual Medicine in
the late 1980s (Kron, 2003:29). Graduates of this program who had studied
osteopathy went on to establish the Australian College of Physical Medicine.
Some members of this association along with the Australian Association of
Musculoskeletal Medicine have adopted chiropractic techniques as well.

While the Australasian College of Nutritional and Environmental
Medicine (ACNEM) does not identify itself as an integrative medicine association per se, many of its members appear to be interested in complementary medicine. This body defines nutritional and environmental medicine
as 'the study of the interactions of both nutritional and environmental factors with human physiology, biochemistry, pathology and anatomy and the
clinical application of these interactions in the optimisation of health and
the prevention and treatment of disease' (www.Nutritional-Environmental-
Medicine.html. Accessed 3/01/2009). ACNEM has collaborated over
the years with the Australasian Integrative Medicine Association, the now
defunct Graduate School of Integrative Medicine at Swinburne University,
and the Australian College of Herbal Medicine. It extends full membership
to biomedical physicians and associate membership to 'registered health
providers with tertiary degrees, such as pharmacists, chiropractors, psychologists, and registered nurses'.

David Mitchell (2008:20) reports that two-thirds of practising biomedical acupuncturists belong to the Australian Medical Acupuncture College, an organisation that was established in 1973 following a visit of a group of Australian biomedical physicians to China where they observed and studied acupuncture. The primary aim of the Australian Medical Acupuncture College is to

> [T]each and continue to educate doctors and dentists in all forms of acupuncture. Training courses are run by state AMAC branches in Queensland and New South and by distance learning through Monash University in Victoria (Mitchell, 2008:20).

The growing interest of biomedical physicians in complementary medicine or integrative medicine is evidenced by three volumes edited by Marc Cohen titled *Prescriptions for Holistic Health* (2002), *Holistic Healthcare in Practice* (2003), and *Holistic Health Perspectives* (2006). Cohen has a biomedical degree from Monash University and training in Traditional Chinese Medicine, is the founding head of the Department of Complementary Medicine at the Royal Melbourne Institute of Technology University, and has served as the president of the Australasian Integrative Medical Association. Cohen also directs the relatively new Master of Wellness Program at RMIT, which is reportedly the first online postgraduate program on wellness (www.rmit.net.au, accessed 5/01/2009).

At any rate, contributors to the three volumes include various biomedical physicians with training in various complementary therapeutic systems. In the case of the second volume, contributors include Tim Bajraszewski, who has a biomedical degree from the University of Melbourne and obtained acupuncture training from the Australian Medical Acupuncture College; Robyn Cosford who has a biomedical degree, studied nutrition, homeopathy, herbalism, Traditional Chinese Medicine, and kinesiology, and established the Northern Beaches Care Centre; and Craig Hassad, who is a general practitioner and senior lecturer at Monash University and has interests in meditation, mind–body medicine, stress management, and counselling.

A prominent contributor to the third volume is Ian Gawler (2006), the founder and director of the Gawler Foundation. While working as a veterinary surgeon, he developed bone cancer, which resulted in the amputation of one of his legs. Shortly thereafter, the cancer returned, prompting Gawler to go on a self-help program consisting of healthy eating, positive thinking, meditation, and compassionate support. He established a cancer support group in 1981 and the Gawler Foundation in 1983. Gawler serves on the advisory board of the Australasian Integrative Medicine Association.

Other contributors to the third volume include Avni Sali, the Foundation Director of the National Institute of Integrative Medicine in Melbourne, and Melvyn A Sydney-Smith, the co-founder in 1980 of the Holistic Medical Centre in Brisbane, the founding director of the Australian College of Holistic Medicine, and an academic staff member in Master of Nutrition Medicine program at the Royal Melbourne Institute of Technology.

As the titles of his three volumes suggest, Cohen seeks to incorporate the notion of holism within integrative medicine. He states,

> [I]ntegrative medicine balances art and science, supportive and cura-
> tive therapies and aims for a true partnership model whereby the prac-
> titioner avoids a paternalistic attitude and fully involves the patient in
> decision making and the implementation of their therapy. In addition,
> the practice of integrative medicine involves principles that can guide
> the implementation of healthcare and base decisions when choos-
> ing between different interventions. These principles include the
> Hippocratic ideal of 'first do no harm', respect for patient autonomy and
> informed consent, as well as consideration of issues of evidence, cost
> effectiveness, practicality, and an awareness that health is influence by
> environmental, physical, emotional and social issues along with spiri-
> tual considerations. When these factors are considered in the full con-
> text of an individual patient's life, the practice can be considered to be
> 'holistic' (Cohen, 2002:7).

The Holistic Health Conference, which started out as the Mind Immunity and Health Conference between 1995 and 1999, has constituted an ongoing effort to incorporate the concept of holism within integrative medicine. The conference initially was sponsored by the Centre for Complementary Medicine at Monash University but later came under the sponsorship of the Australasian Integrative Medicine Association (Cohen, 2002:8, 2004b).

In the United States and Great Britain many biomedical schools now incorporate material on CAM in a variety of venues, including courses that incorporate the expertise of an in-house faculty member, courses that are taught by CAM practitioners from outside the university, courses refer-ring to CAM in the teaching of evidence-based medicine, or courses that involved both biomedical practitioners and CAM practitioners. However, the thirteen Australian biomedical schools have tended to be slow in incor-porating material on complementary medicine (Owen & Lewith, 2004).

Nursing schools in many parts of Australia teach their students vari-ous natural therapies, such as aromatherapy, massage, and Therapeutic Touch (Jacka, 1998:161; Gassib-Spain, Stewart, Tranter, & Young, 2001). The nurs-ing school at the University of Southern Queensland in Toowoomba, for example, has included naturopathy into its curriculum (Eastwood, 1997:20). Pauline McCabe (2001), the editor of *Complementary Therapies in Nursing and Midwifery: From Vision to Practice,* taught naturopathy in the School of Nursing at La Trobe University while the school had a joint nursing–naturopathic program.

The Royal College of Nursing, Australia (RCNA) recognises various complementary therapies that are part and parcel of 'holistic nursing' practice. In its position statement on 'Complementary Therapies in Australian Nursing Practice', it delineates four categories of complementary therapies: (1) 'traditions of healing', such as aromatherapy, acupuncture, and reflexology; (2) 'therapeutic use of self', such as humour, therapeutic touch, and validation therapy; (3) 'physical therapies', such as massage and hydrotherapy; and (4) 'energy therapies', such as meditation, guided imagery, and music therapy. The Royal College states that 'the nursing profession has a responsibility to provide evidence for the efficacy of complementary therapies employed as nursing interventions'.

The Australian College of Holistic Nurses (ACHN) represents nurses committed to 'holistic nursing' and holds annual conferences (www.achn.org.au).

The Australian College of Holistic Nurses has one state association, namely the Holistic Nurses Association of New South Wales (www.achn.org. au/hnansw.htm). It supports the use of complementary therapies in institutional, community, and private health care settings and refers to a wide arrange of modalities, including acupressure, aromatherapy, Bowen technique, flower essences, healing touch, imagery, massage, meditation, natural therapies, reflexology, relaxation, Reiki, shiatsu, Theraepeutic Touch, and visualisation in a booklet on policy guidelines (Australian College of Holistic Nurses, 2000).

Like in North America, many Australians nurses have become involved in energy therapies and touch therapies of various sorts. Two nurses, Mary Jo Bulbrook and Donna Duff, introduced 'healing touch' in a course that they first taught in 1993 (www.healingtouch.org.au, accessed 18/02/2009). The Australian Foundation for Healing Touch represents not only nurses but also complementary practitioners who are interested in this complementary modality (www.healingtouch.org.au).

Holistic nurses in Australia in principle do not wish to adopt complementary therapies as mere adjuncts to biomedical care. Jackie Crisp and Catherine Taylor, two Australian nurses, assert,

> In embracing complementary therapies, nurses need to consider keep-
> ing nursing activity centred on the phenomenon of interpersonal pres-
> ence, or it may eventuate that the therapies become 'quick fix' acts in

themselves, devoid of therapeutic human sensing and presence. In this way, the range of complementary therapies would become little more than a conglomeration of new approaches, applied clinically to certain cases without reference to the unique nature and circumstances of the people concerned (Crisp & Taylor, 2001:983).

In contrast to the principles espoused by Australian holistic nurses, increasingly Australian biomedical physicians are redefining complementary therapeutic systems as modalities within biomedicine or at least closely related to biomedicine. For example, some biomedical general practitioners have come to term chiropractic and osteopathy as physical medicine or manual medicine (Easthope, 1997:14). Dietetics and nutritional advice as treatment modalities integral to naturopathy, homoeopathy, and herbal medicine have been incorporated by biomedical physicians under the designation of nutritional and environmental medicine.

> Acupuncture, in the context of general medical practice, is redefined as medical acupuncture. For example, sports medicine, a group sub-specialty in general practice, relies on remedial therapies that include massage, relaxation and chiropractic and acupuncture techniques... Natural medicine, a more recent term used by orthodox doctors, implies an emphasis on herbs, diet and environment as non-drug and non-invasive healing modes (Easthope, 1997:14).

Obviously, complementary medicine practitioners face competition from biomedical practitioners and nurses who incorporate complementary therapies into their respective practices. Some complementary practitioners maintain that if biomedical practitioners receive Medicare rebates for offering complementary therapies, they should as well be because they have received more extensive training in them. As Hunter observes,

> How should we regard doctors practising natural therapies when most of them have little or no training in these areas? Most have done weekend courses provided by manufacturers or other doctors and their training can only be regarded as incomplete by comparison with professional training in natural therapies. Most natural therapy courses involve some 3 to 4 years of full-time study to complete training in just one discipline (eg, homeopathy, herbal medicine or nutrition)(Hunter, 1997:16).

When asked in an interview for her views about biomedical physicians utilising complementary therapies, Carol Langley, a naturopath replied,

> Bad, because I think it will become a big threat to our profession. I feel slightly offended from being unaccepted by the medical profession over many years, that they are now turning around and using our medicines.

> But more importantly, a naturopathic assessment is time consuming
> and I don't think they have the time to implement it properly (quoted
> in Khoury, 2001b).

Despite the fact that an increasing number of biomedical practitioners
have either adopted a more tolerant attitude toward complementary medicine or have even incorporated complementary therapies into their practices,
a small, but vocal, contingent of critical voices exists with the corridors of
biomedicine. Like the United States, Australia has a biomedical 'skeptics'
or 'quack-watchers' network. John Dwyer, an immunologist and Professor
of Medicine at University of New South Wales appears to be most prominent member of the Australian biomedical skeptics network. He has a long
history of criticising complementary medicine in the media (McCutcheon,
2003). In 1994, Dwyer reportedly participated on the ABC Radio program
'Life Matters' in a debate about biomedical and complementary approaches
to immunisation in which he referred to homoeopathy as the 'most extreme
form of quackery of all the alternative medicines' (quoted in Wearing,
2004:280). He asserts that whereas 'good medicine' assumes an evidence-
based approach to treatment, 'bad medicine' is based on anecdotal evidence
(Dwyer, 2004:647). Dwyer (2004:647) argues that whereas '[g]ood medicine is practised by most orthodox [biomedical] and many complementary
and alternative medicine (CAM) practitioners, [b]ad medicine is practised
by a small number of orthodox and significant number of CAM providers'.
When Bob Carr, Premier of New South Wales, appointed Dwyer to chair
the Health Claims and Consumer Protection Commission, the appointment
was opposed by the 'Complementary Healthcare industry because he allegedly approached Health Funds and requested they discontinue reimbursements for 'unscientific medicine" (The complementary health industry, *Art
of Healing – Byron Bay*, Issue 2:8-9. Autumn 2003).

Many biomedical skeptics are embedded in a nation-wide association
called Australian Skeptics, Incorporated, which defines itself as a 'group
that investigates the paranormal and pseudo-science from a responsible
scientific viewpoint' (Overview of the Skeptics, www.skeptics.com.au/
about/overview.htm, p. 1, accessed 5/11/2008). This organisation has
committees in each of the Australian states and territories and claims to
have some 4,000 members. The Australian Skeptics has published *The
Skeptic*, a quarterly journal, since 1981. In addition to critiquing beliefs
and practices such as alchemy, astrology, parapsychology, New Ageism, the
skeptics attempt to debunk many complementary and alternative systems
or therapies, including acupuncture, Ayurveda, aromatherapy, chiropractic, iridology, naturopathy, Reiki, and Therapeutic Touch, as being 'unscientific', if not fraudulent.

The development of centres of integrative medicine and the growing interest of hospitals and health insurance companies in complementary medicine

Despite the appearance of integrated clinics in Australia, thus far they have not attracted major corporate interest in Australia as they have begun to do so in the United States (Collyer, 2004:89; Easthope, 2004). The Perth Natural Medicine Clinic constitutes an example of an integrative health care centre in Australia. It employs two biomedical physicians, a podiatrist, two osteopaths, four naturopaths, and various other practitioners (Perth Natural Medical Clinic, www.pnmc.com.au/integrativemed.html, accessed 3/9/2004). The Nature Care Holistic and Medical Centre in North Sydney has at its focal point a female general practitioners who reportedly treats about half of the patients, with presumably at least some of these as well as the other patients being treated by 16 complementary practitioners of different sorts (*Insight*, Archives 30 March 2004, www.sbs.com.au/insight). Many Australian pharmacies now offer regular consultation with a complementary therapist, such as a naturopath or homeopath.

Various hospitals have begun to adopt complementary health practices. For example, the Royal Hospital for Women created a Natural Therapies Unit which tests the utility of foods like soy and ginger in treating various ailments (Moynihan, 1999:7). Ramesh Manocha (2001), a biomedical physician, initiated a Meditation Research Program at the same institution. Until its closure in 2005, the Graduate School of Integrative Medicine at Swinburne University offered courses for medical professionals in nutritional and environmental medicine and mind/body medicine and also conducted clinical efficacy trials (Who's Who in the Graduate School of Integrative Medicine, www.swin.edu.au/gsim/gsmednews.html, accessed 30/4/2004). Avni Sali, a surgeon and foundation head of the school, is an honorary patron of the Melbourne Therapy Centre, an Anthroposophy institution. The Graduate School of Integrative Medicine also offered distance education courses for biomedical physicians who wished to incorporate complementary medicine into their practices. Apparently, this program has been replaced by the National Institute of Integrative Medicine, which plans to recommence programmes of study at a site yet to be determined (National Institute of Integrative Medicine, n.d.).

The 60-bed private Swinburne University Hospital in Melbourne offered a wide range of complementary services (Collyer, 2004:89). Furthermore, Shellharbour Private Hospital south of Sydney operates a one-stop medical complex offering both complementary and biomedical services and sells natural and conventional medical products in a facility adjacent to the hospital (Collyer, 2004:89).

Many private insurance companies now reimburse complementary medicine as a marketing strategy for attracting new clients (Collyer, 2004). According to Easthope,

> Those with higher incomes … tend to belong to private health insurance schemes. As Medicare has become more successful, more and more people are withdrawing from such schemes. To capture an increased share of a declining market, the schemes have added various complementary practices to their rebate schedule … For those who cannot afford fees, different forms of complementary health care are available. In particular, the healers who do not charge fees but accept gifts, predominantly religiously based healers, have come into increasing prominence (Easthope, 1993:293).

The natural health products industry–government nexus

Australia has been experiencing a rapid growth in the sale of natural health products over the past several decades. Nevertheless, natural health products have been manufactured and utilised by various types of complementary practitioners for some time in Australia. The natural products industry has literally grown from a cottage industry to a 'mature market sector' (Collyer, 2004:81). These products are sold through retail outlets, including mail order and multi-level marketers and by complementary practitioners, including herbalists and naturopaths, and increasingly biomedical physicians and pharmacies. For example, Discount Natural Health Products (an Australian-based firm) sells a wide range of natural products, including homoeopathics, aromatherapy, natural skin and beauty products, and weight reduction products to customers throughout the world (www.discountnaturalhealth.com, accessed 1/03/2005). The firm offers free naturopathic advice via email communication to potential customers. A 2000 *British Medical Journal* study found the following prevalence rates for utilisation of complementary medicines in their respective general populations: Germany, 65 percent; Canada, 58 percent; France, 50 percent; Australia, 50 percent; United States, 41 percent; Switzerland, 40 percent; Belgium, 30 percent; Sweden, 25 percent; and United Kingdom, 20 percent (www.naturalmedicines.com.au, accessed 3/09/2004). Phillip Daffy (1998:13–14), the Technical Director of Blackmores Ltd. Sydney states: 'A current estimate of wholesale value is that there are approximately AUS$100 million herbal products sold to retailers, and approximately $25 million sales to health professionals, suggesting a total market value of $200 million sales to consumers, given an average 60% markup on wholesale'. Nine large companies produce natural therapies products in Australia and are listed on the Australian Stock Exchange. These are Pan Pharmaceuticals; Faulding, Cenovis, Bullivant (Mayne Group); Clover; Blackmores; Herbs of Gold, Vita Health (Vita Life Sciences); Novogen; Modern Chinese Medicine (Analytica); Pharmacatin, Biologic, BETA (Cottee Health); and Anadis (Collyer, 2004:87). Blackmores, Mediherb, and Cathay Herbal are involved in clinical trials. Australian Tea Tree Oil Research Institute is situated at SCU (Daffy, 1998:15). Much mainstreaming of natural products industry in Australia has occurred 'through mergers and acquisitions rather than by companies altering their manufacturing processes or internally expanding their product line through R&D' (Collyer, 2004:90). Pharmaceutical companies have entered the natural products industry by either introducing natural medicines into their own range of products or purchasing smaller companies that manufacture these products. In 1999, for example, Faulding took over the two largest Australian natural products manufacturers (Sherwood, 2004:225). The pharmaceutical industry enjoys considerable influence in Australia, despite the fact that only pharmaceuticals manufactured in Australia are made under license. It has managed to obtain places on the board of the Pharmaceuticals Benefit Scheme which assesses efficacy of prescription drugs (Easthope, 2004:323).

The pricing and regulation of both prescription drugs and natural products has been a political football in Australia as well as across the globe. According to Whyte, van der Geest, and Hardon,

> In practice, policy making and implementation are influenced by networks of global and national planners, scientists, industry representatives, activists, Non-Governmental Organizations, and public and private donors. And the policies are affected by globalization processes that undermine the implementation of equity-oriented public health policies. These processes include the increased privatisation of health care services, and the implementation of liberalized trade policies that define medicines as commercial goods, protected by intellectual rights (Whyte, van der Geest, & Hardon, 2002:148).

In 1981, the Food Standards Committee collaborated with the National Health and Medical Research Council in the drafting of standards designed to restrict the administration of vitamins and mineral preparations to biomedical physicians (Brownie, 2005:194). Upon receiving some 250,000 letters of protest against the proposed measure, the Federal government withdrew it from further consideration.

The Therapeutic Goods Act of 1989, which was first implemented in 1991, is designed to 'ensure the quality, safety and efficacy of therapeutic goods available to the Australian public, so that consumers can have confidence in the medicines available to them' (Cummings, 2000:57). The Therapeutic Goods Administration regulates both pharmaceuticals and natural medicinal products in Australia. The Act 'replaced the state and territory-based regulatory structures with a uniform, national set of statutory guidelines for the import, export, manufacture and supply of medicines in Australia' (Brownie, 2005:197). As a result of the new federal regulatory structure, some small natural products manufacturers, such as Greenpharm, had to cease operations because of their inability to meet the expense of regulatory compliance (Canaway, 2007).

The previous Liberal–National Coalition government had promised easier access to complementary medicines and has been critical of biomedicine for restrictive practices that purportedly disadvantage health consumers. The Alternative Medicine Summit held in Old Parliament House on 16 October 1996 and the Therapeutic Goods Administration Review constitute examples of the Government's commitment to complementary medicine regulatory reform. Goods that are classified as *registered* (eg, prescription drugs) are required to exhibit quality, safety, and efficacy. *Listed goods*, such as vitamins and suntan lotions) are required to exhibit only quality and safety but not efficacy.

In 1997, the federal government created the Complementary Medicines Evaluation Committee which was mandated with the role of evaluating and reporting on the registration or listing of natural products. This committee includes representatives from the natural products industry, consumer groups, and government agencies (Natural Medicine Industry, www.naturalmedicines.com.au, accessed 3/09/2004, p. 2). The inclusion of industry parties within the TGA supports the assertion on the part of 'capture theorists' that regulatory bodies often become biased in favour of industrial interests, despite initial assertions that the regulatory body was created in order to protect the public interest (Abraham, 1995:22–23).

Senator Trambling created the Working Party on Complementary Medicines within the TGA on 2 December 1998 for the purpose of developing regulatory reforms aimed to 'provide more transparent and efficient market access to complementary healthcare products while maintaining the current high standards of public health and safety regulation' (Khoury, 1999). About 40 delegates attended briefings. The Commonwealth implemented the Complementary Medicines Reform Package in 1999 that included the creation of the Office of Complementary Medicine as a component of the TGA, the enhancement of the Complementary Medicines Evaluation Committee, and the creation of the establishment of the Complementary Healthcare Consultative Forum, an industry/government body (NSWHEALTH, 2002:9). While complementary medicines or natural products in theory can be classified as either listed or registered, they generally fall under the listed designation.

Australia has become one of the few Anglophone countries regulating herbal preparations as registered medicines. Some worry that the herbal product industry is becoming too 'phytomedicinal' as pharmaceutical companies become more interested in marketing herbal products (Daffy, 1998:14). Evans (2000a:21) argues that the Therapeutic Goods Act has contributed to the demise of small natural medicine products manufacturers with only the medium to large-scale businesses being able to survive.

Like other Australian universities that have come to increasingly enter into partnerships with various industries, Southern Cross University has become involved in efficacy testing of various natural products. It is now a leading force in promoting research on herbal medicine in Australia. SCU sponsored the 'Herbal Medicine into the New Millennium' conference 16–18 June 1999 which had developed out of the Cellulose Valley project at the university (Fechter et al., 1999). The conference involved 27 keynote speakers and poster sessions that provided a venue for industry specialists and students to display their research. Peter Baverstock (1999:iii), Dean of Research, at SCU observed: 'We wanted the conference to be in keeping with the Cellulose Valley theme – that of creating synergies between scientists and researchers, manufacturers, primary producers, regulators, and of course practitioners of herbal medicine'.

Howard Rubin (1999:11–14) noted that the Northern Rivers Herb Growers Association was formed by 15 people in 1987. This body grew to include about 100 members by 1990, changed its name to Organic Herb Growers of Australia Inc, and came to have a national membership of 580 with 350 certified organic farms representing some 1,000 hectares of production, most in herbs (Rubin, 1999:11). A larger project entailing an industry partnership with Southern Cross University is the Cellulose Valley Institute which claims to be the 'world's most comprehensive plant research collective' (www.cellulosevalley.com, p. 1, accessed 21/01/2005). Its products are tested at the Southern Cross University naturopathic clinic and the University of Queensland's clinical facilities in Brisbane.

The TGA learned that some 80 individuals who had taken Travacalm (a travel sickness preventive medicine manufactured by Pan Pharmeuticals), 19 of who had to be hospitalised, had developed negative side-effects (TGA Expert Committee on Complementary Medicines in the Health System, www.health.gov.au/tga/docs/html/cmreport.htm, accessed 29/04/2004; *Skeptical Inquirer,* 2003:1–2). The agency conducted an analysis of Travacalm purchased from a pharmacy that indicated that the tablets in one package contained amounts of active ingredient, hyoscine, varying between none at all and seven times the safe dosage. The TGA audited the company and discovered serious quality control problems. It recalled over 1,500 complementary medicines from the Australian market in April 2003 and evoked Pan's manufacturing license. The TGA exempted Pan-produced prescription drugs that fell under the Pharmaceutical Benefits Scheme from the recall because they had been subjected to a safety assessment (McGregor, 2003–2004:20).

Pan had supplied 75 percent of Australia's complementary healthcare products, including nutritional supplements in the form of vitamins, minerals, omega oils, and other drugs. It also supplied a range of over-the-counter drugs and prescription drugs, which were sold under various brand names by other companies. Pan was founded and owned by Jim Selim, an Egyptian-born pharmacist. He transformed the company into the largest supplier of natural products in Australia and the fourth largest manufacturer of natural health products in the world (Hillary, Eve. Part 1 – Pan, www.livingnow. com.au/issues, accessed 11/11/2004, p. 1). Pan claimed that one of its analysts was responsible for a lapse in quality control over the defective product that resulted in his firing.

In May 2004, the Australian government formed the Expert Committee on Complementary Medicines in the Health System to guarantee Australia's reputation as a supplier of high quality and safe medicines (Department of Health and Ageing, Therapeutic Goods Administration, Expert Committee on Complementary Medicines in the Health System, 2003). Membership consisted of 18 members, including Dr. Michael Bollen (Chair), a former member of National Health and Medical Research Council; Alan Bensoussan; Stephen Myers; David McLeod, a representative of the Australian Acupuncture and Chinese Medicine Association; and Darrin Walters, CEO, Blackmores Ltd. The Australian government's rationale for health policy reforms in complementary medicine stresses consumer choice and empowerment by promoting increased knowledge, product safety, and proven efficacy through government regulation of industry. Within the rubric of complementary medicines, the Expert Committee (2003:43) includes 'herbal medicines, vitamin and mineral supplements, other nutritional supplements, traditional medicines such as Ayurvedic medicines and Traditional Chinese Medicines (TCM), homeopathic medicines, and aromatherapy oils'. The Committee recommended that the enhanced training for all practitioners who prescribe or advice on the use of complementary medicines should be strengthened and encouraged and called for increased government funding for complementary medicines research.

To date the Australian government has been slow to fund research on complementary medicine. Bensoussan and Lewith (2004:331) report that 'only $850,000 of about $1 billion of National Health and Medical Research Council (NHMRC) research funding has been allocated to CAM research in total in Australia since 2001'. Victoria has provided a seed grant of $500,000 for the creation of an Australian Research Centre for Complementary and Alternative Medicines. Conversely, the natural products industry has tended to be reluctant to invest in efficacy research rather than marketing, in large part because it lacks a research tradition.

Various organisations have sought to legitimise the natural products industry through public relations and lobbying the federal government. According to Brownie,

> The natural therapies profession played a significant role in the development of dietary supplement policies in this country. In Australia, representatives from this profession have been instrumental in mobilising public interest in this topic and in determining the outcome of legislation affecting access to dietary supplements (Brownie, 2005:193–194).

The Complementary Healthcare Council, based in Canberra, represents the complementary health industry in Australia (Johanson, 1999). In 2004, its executive committee included six suppliers, three retailers, one healthcare professional, and one consumer (Complementary Healthcare Council – Structure, www.chc.org/au, p. 1, accessed 8/04/2004).

The Natural Health Care Alliance (est. 2003) seeks funds for a campaign to counteract alleged negativity and media bias against 'Natural Healthcare Industry and promotes freedom of choice of healthcare (www.nhca.com. au, accessed 21/03/2004). NHCA aims to 'provide a single voice for all of these professional groups in complementary medicine, and a vehicle for their participation in political and regulatory areas relevant to their modality or expertise' (Natural Health Care Alliance, 2004:7). Its steering committee includes Dr. Mark Donohue, Daniel Baden (TMS & Vitasearch), Rod Brennan (Nature Care College), Russell Norden (*Journal of Complementary Medicine*), Dr. Karen Bridgman, and Patricia Reed, RN. NHCA prefers the term 'natural healthcare' over 'complementary medicine' which it asserts 'has the effect of prejudicing a debate, suggesting similarity to medicine where little similarity exists' (National Health Care Alliance, 2004:13). It maintains that 'truly effective and sustainable health care is best achieved by an open, competitive market and even playing field in terms of subsidies and taxes, and that the health of Australians is currently placed at risk by Government support for a medical monopoly which consumes ever increasing resources with no evidence of improved outcomes or benefits to the consumer' (Natural Health Care Alliance, 2004:15).

The Australian Committee of Natural Therapies claims to represent 'Natural, Traditional, Bioenergetic and Magnetic Therapies' and the 'manufacturers, importers, suppliers, and also the practitioners, of complementary and alternative medical therapy and testing devices' (www.acont.org. au, accessed 6/11/2008).

The TGA has been criticised by representatives of both biomedicine and the natural products industry. John Dwyer, Australia's leading biomedical skeptic, asserts,

> The TGA's current approach seems to be determined by resource issues rather than any proof that its procedures adequately protect consumers. At the moment, the proponents of products listed with the TGA are told that they must keep on record proof of the efficacy of any claims made, and that significant penalties will be applied if the TGA ever finds that such evidence was not available. The TGA carries out random checks, but the system is manifestly inadequate (Dwyer, 2004:648).

Conversely, Marcus C. Blackmore (n.d.:3), a leading natural products manufacturer, argues that the TGA is 'stifled by a pharma mindset'. Indeed, TGA representatives, along with representatives from the US Food and Drug Administration regularly attend meetings of the Codex Alimentarius Commission that meets once a year in a European city (Hillary, Eve – Part 1 – Pan, p. 6). The Commission reportedly consists primarily of representatives from large multinational companies and government drug regulating authorities. It does not include representatives from small vitamin manufacturers and retailers and has increasingly come to classify herbs as drugs with restricted access. At any rate, Blackmore urged Parliamentary Secretary Senator Chris Ellison to create the Complementary Medicines Evaluation Committee in order to address concerns within the natural products industry concerning an allegedly pro-pharmaceutical industry bias and called for the removal of Val Johanson from the position of Executive Director of the Complementary Healthcare Council and Joachim Fluhrer, an integrative medicine practitioner, from membership in the Council (Blackmore n.d.:7). Blackmore recommended the establishment of a new Complementary Medicines Advisory Committee. Sue Evans (2000a:21), a herbalist and naturopath, argues that while the Therapeutic Goods Act granted natural medicine products with a certain legitimacy by defining them 'legally, on the statute books, as therapeutic', it has contributed to the demise of their production as a cottage industry.

Barry Williams (2003), the CEO of the Australian Skeptics, argues that the alleged relaxation of governmental regulations for natural health products has contributed to a rapid increase in their sale. He suggests that his organisation helped to short-circuit an effort on the part of the Complementary Healthcare Council to obtain a $11 million grant to fund public education on the benefits of natural health products and commends the TGA on its crack-down of Pan Pharmaceuticals and the federal government's promotion of legislation requiring a higher degree of compliance, proof of efficacy, and accuracy of labelling of natural products.

Summary

In response to the holistic health movement and the widespread popularity of complementary medicine in Australia, over the past three decades or so a growing number of Australian biomedical physicians and nurses have become interested in complementary medicine. Increasingly, Australian biomedical physicians are redefining complementary therapies as modalities within biomedicine or at least closely related to biomedicine. Despite efforts on the proponents of holistic health and complementary medicine to develop an alternative to biomedicine, what in reality have been in Australia the beginnings of the co-option of complementary medicine under the rubric of integrative medicine. Nurses have been less a part of the co-optive process in part due to their subservient status vis-à-vis biomedical physicians. On another plane, in reality, many Australians rely not so much on complementary practitioners as they do on complementary medicines or natural products that have in the past been produced by small natural products firms. However, just as biomedical practitioners are being impacted by larger health structures, both public and private, the natural products industry is being increasingly dominated and even absorbed by the larger pharmaceutical industry.

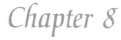

Chapter 8

An overview of complementary medicine in New Zealand

Introduction

In contrast to Australia where the term *complementary medicine* is widespread, in New Zealand the terms *complementary and alternative medicine* (CAM) or *complementary and alternative health* (CAH) are commonplace. The New Zealand Charter of Health Practitioners (est. 1993) estimates that there were about 10,000 CAH practitioners in New Zealand in 2001, with some 8,500 of them being represented by the Charter (New Zealand Health Workforce, 2001:176). The Charter represents 68 associations. At any rate, according to anthropologist Philippa Ann Miskelly,

> Despite the early obstacles practitioners faced in establishing and prac-
> ticing alternative and complementary medicines, these are now well
> established in New Zealand and are part of a burgeoning health care
> industry. Patients can access a veritable smorgasbord of CAM therapies
> such as radionic and psionic medicine, colour therapy, herbal medi-
> cine, naturopathy, homeopathy and Bach flower remedies through to
> practices involving spiritual surgery or attendance at New Age aware-
> ness retreats (Miskelly, 2006:123).

Various studies have indicated extensive patient utilisation of CAM thera-
pies in New Zealand (Dixon et al., 1977; Leibrich, Hickling, and Pitt, 1987; McIver, 1997; Ministry of Health, 1997; New Zealand Consumers' Institute, 1997). As noted earlier, the 2002/2003 New Zealand Survey provides provisional results in terms of the number of New Zealand adults who visited a CAM practitioner at least once during a 12-month period. Table 21 summarises the findings of the survey.

The New Zealand dominative medicine

Like other state societies, New Zealand has a dominative medical system which is depicted in Figure 2. Chiropractic and osteopathy constitute the only CAM systems that have achieved statutory registration, a scenario similar to that in Australia, with the exception of Chinese medicine which achieved statutory registration in Victoria in 2000.

CAM practitioner visited	Consumers as % of NZers	Female consumers as % of females interviewed	Male consumers as % of males interviewed
All CAM practitioners	23.4	28.1	18.4
Massage therapist	9.1	11.6	6.4
Chiropractor	6.1	6.3	6.0
Osteopath	4.9	6.1	3.6
Homeopath or naturopath	4.5	6.8	1.9
Acupuncturist	2.6	3.4	1.9
Spiritual healer	1.9	2.3	1.5
Herbalist	1.8	2.5	1.0
Traditional Chinese Medicine	1.4	1.9	0.7
Maori healer	0.9	1.0	0.7
Pacific healer	0.2	0.3	0.2
Feldernkrais or Alexander technique	0.2	0.2	–
Aromatherapist	0.7	1.0	0.4
Other practitioners	1.3	1.5	0.9

*Adapted from ministerial advisory committee on complementary and alternative health (2004:67)

Figure 2
The New
Zealand
dominative
medical system

Biomedicine
Fully legitimised heterodox medical systems
    Chiropractic
    Osteopathy
Partially legitimised heterodox medical systems
    Naturopathy
    Chinese medicine and acupuncture
    Homeopathy
    Massage therapy
Marginal heterodox medical systems
    Reiki, Shiatsu, reflexology
Religious healing systems
    Christian science
    Spiritualism
    Pentecostalism
    Scientology
    New Age medicine
Folk medical systems
    Pakeha folk medicine
    Maori folk medicine
    South Pacific Islander folk medicine
    Asian folk medical systems: Chinese, Korean, Indian, etc

Chiropractic in New Zealand

Chiropractic entered New Zealand around World War I (Duke, 2005). Despite the fact that most early New Zealand chiropractors were graduates of the Palmer School of Chiropractic, the first of the chiropractic colleges and a bastion of straight chiropractic, the New Zealand Chiropractic Association (NZCA), attempted to stay clear of the disputes between the straight and mixer chiropractic schools in the United States (Reader & Bryner, 1989). Conversely, it tended to align itself with the straight-oriented International Chiropractic Association and distance itself from the mixer-oriented National Chiropractic Association, which had sent Dr. Nugent to speak at the NZCA conference in 1955. The NZCA played an active role in the establishment of the International College of Chiropractic in Australia.

The Chiropractors Act of 1960 required applicants to have a university degree or its equivalent in the form of a certificate, diploma, or degree or license from an institution which was recognised by the New Zealand Chiropractic Board (Commission of Inquiry, 1979:69). As chiropractors grew in number, they encountered increasing opposition from biomedicine but apparently never on the scale that they had historically experienced in the United States (Baer, 2001:67–84). Beginning in the 1960s, the *New Zealand Medical Journal* published editorials and letters commenting upon chiropractic, generally in a critical manner (Dew, 2003:42). According to Dew,

> In 1975 the medical profession was stirred into outright condemnation of chiropractic when the Petitions Committee of the New Zealand House of Representatives received submissions on a petition [containing 94,210 signatures] to amend the Social Securities Act 1964 and the Accident compensation Act 1972. These amendments would have allowed chiropractors to receive state benefits and their patients to be compensated for the cost of chiropractic treatment in cases of personal injury (Dew, 2003:42).

Chiropractic achieved statutory recognition in New Zealand as a result of the implementation of recommendations made by the Commission of Inquiry into Chiropractic in the late 1970s, thus enabling it to overcome its marginality under Common Law (Dew, 2003:42–56). Two earlier commission investigations had been conducted on the question as to whether chiropractic treatment should be covered under governmental health benefits (Committee of Inquiry, 1979:7). The Royal Commission on Compensation for Personal Injury and later the Royal Commission on Social Security declined to reach a definitive decision on this matter without further biomedical and scientific evidence supporting it. In the process of achieving some semblance of legitimation, the New Zealand Chiropractic Association distanced itself from D.D. Palmer's assertion that subluxations are the sources of most diseases and presented its practitioners as musculoskeletal specialists rather than drugless general practitioners (Dew, 2003).

The New Zealand College of Chiropractic was established in 1994 in Auckland by the New Zealand Chiropractors Association (www.nzchiro. co.nz). It recently moved to a new campus in the Auckland suburb of Mt. Wellington and is accredited by the Council on Chiropractic Education Australasia.

Osteopathy in New Zealand

Despite the fact that chiropractic developed some two decades or so later than osteopathy in the United States, the latter appeared later than chiropractic in New Zealand, reportedly in the early 1930s (Duke, 2005). Osteopaths in New Zealand in the past obtained their training in Britain, Australia, and possibly elsewhere. The New Zealand Registered of Osteopaths was created in 1973 and 'grew steadily for the next five years when it was realized that some form of legislation would be required' (Duke, 2005).

Various osteopathic bodies reportedly asked to be included in this parliamentary inquiry but the Commission of Inquiry in the late 1970s, while recognising similarities between chiropractic and osteopathy, decided not to do so on the grounds that it would have 'substantially protracted' the investigation (Commission of Inquiry, 1979:7). New Zealand chiropractors obtained 'statutory regulation' under the provisions of the Chiropractors Act, 1982.

Like in Australia, New Zealand osteopathy appears to have been riding the political coattails of chiropractic, although not quite to the same extent thus far. After a prolonged lobbying process, New Zealand osteopaths finally obtained statutory registration when osteopathy was included under the provisions of the Health Practitioners Competence Act, 2003 which came into law on 18 September 2004 and repealed the eleven previously existing health occupation regulatory statutes, including the Chiropractors Act, 1982 (www.osteopathiccouncil.org.nz). The Osteopathic Council of New Zealand regulates the osteopathic profession.

The Osteopathic Society of New Zealand represents members in negotiations and interactions with various bodies, including governmental health bodies, private health insurance companies, the Osteopathic Council of New Zealand, and the Australian Osteopathic Association.

The Accident Compensation Corporation, a government scheme, subsidises not only chiropractic but also osteopathy and acupuncture services offered by certain providers. Work and Income New Zealand pays a disability allowance to cover the cost of complementary medicine treatment offered by chiropractors, osteopaths, biomedical practitioners practicing acupuncture and homeopathy, and physiotherapists practicing acupuncture.

Since February 2002, UNITEC in Auckland has been offering a five-year Master of Osteopathy degree that allows individuals to register with the Osteopathic Council of New Zealand (www.unitec.ac.nz). Growing interest on the part of biomedicine in manual medicine is evidenced by the fact that the Department of Orthopaedic Surgery and Musculoskeletal Medicine at the Christchurch School of Medicine offers a postgraduate certificate in Musculoskeletal Medicine that includes training in chiropractic and osteopathy (University of Otago, 2002).

Whereas in the United States insurance companies, Medicare (the federal health plan for people over age 65) and Medicaid (the federal health plan for the indigent poor) cover services provided by osteopathic physicians, the governments of Australia, New Zealand as well as Britain and Canada provide some but limited financial reimbursements for osteopathic services. In contrast to the United States where osteopathy or osteopathic medicine and chiropractic have evolved in quite different directions, osteopathy shares roughly the same niche as chiropractic in the medical marketplaces of Australia and New Zealand, again along with Britain and Canada. Although osteopathy in Canada, Britain, and Australasia tends to resemble what it looked like 80 or 90 years ago in the United States, it also has, like chiropractic, been partially medicalised in these settings as it has embarked upon a path of professionalisation and legitimisation.

In contrasting their philosophy to the reductionist one of biomedical physicians, many osteopaths claim that they practice a holistic form of health care which focuses upon the treatment of the whole person. In the United States, osteopathic physicians frequently assert that they treat the person rather than the disease. However, in reality this assertion still requires empirical proof. In reality, there are various philosophical orientations within osteopathy. William Garner Sutherland (1873–1954), a student of Andrew Taylor Still, developed cranial osteopathy, a system premised upon the notion that the manipulation of the cranial bones could correct a variety of physical and psychological complications. In the 1930s he began to postulate that the tissues, organs, and bones of the cranium exhibit a dynamic state of motion. Indeed, Sutherland attributed a 'vitality to the CSF [cranial sacral fluid], endowing it with mystical if not spiritual qualities, much as blood had been endowed by earlier generations' (Harries, 2000:144). In large part, however, osteopathy, has increasingly sought validation by relying upon evidence-based medicine and randomised, double-blind, controlled trials as is evident in most of the publications in the *International Journal of Osteopathic Medicine*. In reality, like biomedicine, the holism of osteopathy tends to be limited in that it relies heavily on notions such as the machine analogy and osteopathic lesions as the cause of disease. Indeed, McQueen discusses the similarities of biomedicine or allopathy, osteopathy, and chiropractic:

> The body is viewed as a machine, in some cases a god-given perfect machine, in other cases a chemical–physical machine. In both cases the body is seen as normally running without trouble: occasionally, however, it needs repair or adjustment. Chiropractic and osteopathic concern themselves with the structure and function of the machine. Healing occurs by making structural corrections ... Allopathic doctrines concern themselves with how the machine has been damaged by foreign parts, either injury, tumors, germs, or other invaders (McQueen, 1978:74).

Furthermore, allopathy, osteopathy, and chiropractic, at least in their original form, imply that healing involves the removal of single cause: a pathogen in the case of allopathy, a lesion in the case of osteopathy, and a subluxation in the case of chiropractic.

Naturopathy and the natural therapies in New Zealand

Unlike chiropractic and osteopathy, all other CAM medical systems lack statutory registration in New Zealand. Naturopathy and the natural therapies in New Zealand are represented by a large number of associations and colleges, albeit not to the same extent as in Australia, not surprising given that New Zealand has about one-fifth the population of its huge neighbour across the Tasman Sea.

The New Zealand Charter of Health Practitioners (est. 1993) is the largest CAM umbrella organisation in New Zealand (www.healthcharter.org. nz, accessed 3/5/2007). Another similar body is the New Zealand Register of Complementary Health Professionals. The Natural Health Council (NZ) evolved from the NZ Natural Health Practitioners Accreditation Board (est. 1987) to create education standards for naturopathy, homeopathy, herbal medicine, remedial body therapies, and osteopathy (www.naturalhealth-council.org.nz, accessed 3/05/2007). This body reportedly has 112 registered members in New Zealand and seven overseas. The New Zealand Natural Medicine Association seeks to integrate biomedical and CAM modalities in New Zealand (www.nznma.com, accessed 29/06/2007).

The New Zealand Society of Naturopaths admits for membership graduates of the South Pacific College of Natural Therapeutics, the Naturopathic College of New Zealand, and the Wellpark College of Natural Therapies as well as graduates from other colleges who can demonstrate proof that they have completed 300 hours of nutrition, 300 hours of anatomy and physiology, 125 hours of pathology, 400 hours of herbs/homeopathy, 250 hours of remedial body therapy, 125 hours of diagnostics, 50 hours of counseling, 200 hours of clinical practice, 100 hours of biochemistry, 100 hours of pharmacological drugs, and 50 hours of law and ethics (www.naturopath.org.nz). The New Zealand Charter Practitioners Incorporated (est. 1993) based in Auckland represents various natural therapists (www.healthcharter.org.nz, accessed 10/06/2005).

The New Zealand Natural Medicine Association is dedicated to integrative medicine, an effort to blend biomedicine and complementary and alternative medicine. It offers associate membership to registered health providers with tertiary training such as pharmacists, chiropractors, psychologists, and RNs (www.nznma.com). The association counts naturopaths, herbalists, osteopaths, herbalists, and biomedical physicians among its members.

The New Zealand Association of Medical Herbalists was established in the 1930s and merged in 2000 with the Aotearoa Herbalists Incorporated, a body created by students at the Waikato Centre for Herbal Studies in 1994. NZAMH has four categories of members: (1) 'Professional Members who have graduated from Herbal Medicine courses at colleges approved by NZAMH or else have passed examinations set by the New Zealand Natural Health Practitioners Accreditation Board and have completed 100 clinic hours with a recognised Herbal College'; (2) student members; (3) 'Associate members are individuals or groups involved in some aspect of medicinal herbs, for example, growing, producing, or promoting medicinal herbs;' and (4) 'Fellow members are elected by the association to honour members who have given conspicuous service'. The association has local meetings in Auckland, Whangarei, Hamilton-Cambridge-Raglan Tauranga and Nelson.

There are numerous schools that offer programs of study in naturopathy and the natural therapies scattered about New Zealand (see Appendix 6). According to Miskelly,

> The training of some CAM practitioners is becoming more *mainstream*. This is because an increasing number of institutions are offering courses that include a biomedical component, such as papers [subjects or courses] on anatomy or pharmaceutical interactions. Some of my participants believed this will bolster public and biomedical confidence in the sector because practitioners who do not meet required standards will not be eligible for inclusion on therapeutic registers and this may eventually force them out of business (Miskelly, 2006:169).

The Naturopathic College of New Zealand was established in 1979 by Melva Martin and is situated in New Plymouth on the North Island (www. naturopathycollege.com). It encourages its graduates to join an association that is affiliated with the New Zealand Charter of Health Practitioners. This institution has been receiving Ministry of Education funding for courses since 1998 and offers the Diploma of Naturopathy, the Diploma of Remedial Body Therapies, the National Diploma of Reflexology, the National Diploma of Aromatherapy, and the National Diploma of Massage Therapy, and various certificates.

The Wellpark College of Natural Therapies in Auckland offers diploma programs in naturopathy and herbal medicine, massage and aromatherapy, and Ayurvedic medicine yoga (www.wellpark.co.nz, accessed 10/06/2008). The Diploma of Naturopathy entails three years of full-time study but may be pursued on a part-time basis. Graduates of the naturopathic program may obtain an additional diploma in Herbal Medicine and/or Nutrition by taking additional course work.

The Canterbury College of Natural Medicine (est. 1994) is located in Christchurch and claims to be the 'leading education provider of natural/ alternative medicine on the South Island'. It offers diplomas in massage therapy and clinical nutrition and a graduate diploma in nutrition medicine (www.ccnm.ac.nz, accessed 29/06/2007). The South Pacific College of Natural Therapeutics offers Advanced Diploma in Naturopathy plus/or an Advanced Diploma in Herbal Medicine that can lead to the Bachelor of Health Science (Complementary Medicine) at Charles Sturt University in Australia (www.spcnt.ac.nz). The Lotus Holistic Centre offers diplomas in naturopathy and herbal medicine (www.lotusmassage.co.nz).

Natural therapies are also taught at various other institutions. Aoraki Polytechnic offers a certificate in Complementary Therapies; Auckland University of Technology a certificate in Holistic Therapies; and Otago Polytechnic a certificate in Massage Therapy. It operates a clinic and offers a one-year full-time course in medical herbalism (www.ccnm.ac.nz).

Chinese medicine and acupuncture in New Zealand

Like in Australia, the first practitioners of Chinese medicine and acupuncture in New Zealand were Chinese immigrants who arrived in the late nineteenth and early twentieth centuries (Duke, 2005). The New Zealand Acupuncture Society (est. 1975) appears to be the earliest association representing Chinese medicine practitioners and acupuncturists. The New Zealand Register of Acupuncturists was established in 1977 (Duke, 2005). The New Zealand Institute of Acupuncture reportedly consists of biomedical physicians, nurses, physiotherapists, osteopaths, chiropractors, and Chinese medicine practitioners (The New Zealand Health Workforce, 2001:178).

The New Zealand School of Acupuncture and TCM (est. 1989) has campuses in Auckland and Wellington and claims to be the largest Chinese medicine school in the country (www.acupuncture.co.nz, accessed 3/05/2007). It offers a Diploma in Acupuncture and Chinese Herbal Medicine and a Diploma in Tuina-Qigong.

The New Zealand College of Chinese Medicine is situated in Christchurch and Auckland and offers diplomas in Traditional Chinese Medicine, Chinese herbal medicine, acupuncture and Tui Na (www.newzealand.govt.nz, accessed 3/05/2007). This institution was formed as a merger in 2006 of the Auckland College of Natural Medicine and the Christchurch College of Holistic Healing (est. 1999).

Homeopathy in New Zealand

The New Zealand Council of Homoeopaths functions largely as an informational body for laypeople interested in homeopathy, maintains a registry of practitioners, and conducts monthly meetings in Auckland (www.homoeopathica.org.nz, accessed 3/05/2007). Alfred G. Grove, a homeopath, created the organisation in 1951. There are three part-time homeopathic colleges in New Zealand, namely the Wellington College of Homoeopathy, the Bay of Plenty College of Homoeopathy, and the Auckland College of Classical Homeopathy. The Bay of Plenty College of Homeopathy offers a Diploma and an Advanced Diploma in Homeopathy, a Homoeopathy Foundation course, and a Diploma in Aromatherapy.

Other partially professionalised CAM systems in New Zealand

Unfortunately, relatively little information is available on various other partially professionalised heterodox or CAM medical systems in New Zealand. Appendix 5, however, indicates that numerous small associations and schools representing body workers, reflexologists, hypnotherapists, and other types of CAM practitioners exist in New Zealand. An example of such associations is the Therapeutic Massage Association (est. 1989) and an example of such schools is the Aromaflex International Aromatherapy School which offers an Advanced Certificate in Reflexology, a Diploma in Reflexology, and a subject on 'Introduction to Reflexology'.

Religious and folk medical systems in New Zealand

Maori medicine is the best researched of the various religious and folk medical systems found in New Zealand. Unfortunately, other religious and ethnic folk medical systems in New Zealand, such as Pakeha, Chinese, Korean, or Indian, appear to have received either no or little scholarly attention.

Traditional Maori healing incorporates the use of medicinal plants or herbal remedies (*rongoa*), massage (*mirimiri*), prayer (*karakia*), and other healing rituals. According to Quinn,

> Maori healing differs from conventional medicine in several ways. The person is treated holistically, and not solely for the ailment with which they present. Many factors are examined to try to determine the cause or recurrence of illness, particularly lifestyle, diet, and psychological factors such as stress, anxiety, or depression (Quinn, 2006:5).

The *tohunga* (meaning 'skilled person') is the primary traditional Maori healer. He encompasses various roles: diviner; ritual specialist in terms of activities associated with hunting, fishing, horticultural, navigation, war, birth, marriage, and illness, and death (Lange, 1999:12). After European contact, some *tohungas* supplemented their use of herbal medicine with Western patent remedies and even alcohol (Lange, 1999:48). The persistence of both local and iterant traditional healers prompted colonial and government authorities to characterise them as charlatans and quacks, resulting in the passage of the Tohunga Suppression Act in 1907. However, as Lange (1999:255) observes, '[w]illingness to consult a tohunga has persisted to this day'.

Indeed, traditional Maori has undergone a revival under the manner of Maori nationalism over the course of the past several decades. According to Durie,

> There are a number of reasons why Maori interest in traditional healing has increased. These include the removal of legal barriers following the repeal of the Tohunga Suppression Act in 1964, a greater desire for autonomy and self-determination, the limitations of biomedical methods at least in failing to make serious impact on lifestyle disorders, difficulties accessing the conventional health care system, and a desire to address spiritual causes of poor health (Durie, 2001:161)

In 1995, the Central Regional Health Authority signed with Te Whare Whakapikiora o te Rangimarie for the provision of traditional Maori medicine healing services. An evaluation of the service indicated high utilisation, with over 200 cases being registered over the course of the first six months and a total of 1,766 cases being registered at the time of the study (Lawson-Te Aho, 1996). A study conducted by the Women's Welfare League found that approximately one-fifth of the 1,177 interviews indicated willingness to visit a traditional Maori if one were readily available (Murchie, 1984). A study of

397 Maori over age 60 revealed that 13 percent had visited a Maori healer in the past year and 19 percent expressed preference for a Maori healer if one were available (Te Pumanawa Haoura, 1997).

Maori healing services are funded by the Ministry of Health under the terms of the Treaty of Waitangi. Durie (2001:157) delineates three Maori healing approaches: (1) traditional healing which relies primarily on customary practices; (2) bicultural ones in which Maori healers, psychologists, and counsellors work in partnerships with biomedical or Western health services; and (3) 'Maori-centred approaches' in which Maori values and beliefs serve as the primary basis for treatment. Maori-centred therapies have developed as a response to the perceived inadequacies of bicultural approaches. According to Durie, Maori-centred therapists

> allow clients to work through their own needs, but they supply knowl-
> edge and supply knowledge and perspective and use a variety of songs,
> stories, traditions and physical therapies such as dance. Mauri therapy
> aims to foster a stronger cultural identity and to restore a sense of
> vitality and purpose within the rubric of traditional knowledge. The
> underlying premise is that the acquisition of traditional values and
> beliefs will improve mental health and lead to better adjustment in
> contemporary activities (Durie, 2001:169).

Traditional Maori health clinics are principally designed for use by Indigenous people but may be accessed by people of other ethnic backgrounds. The clinics also collaborate with biomedical practitioners, physiotherapists, Chinese medicine practitioners and acupuncturists, and massage therapists (Quinn, 2006:6). The number of Maori healers increased between 1993 and 2000 from about 20 to 220 (Dew, 2003:115).

Interest of New Zealand biomedicine and nursing in CAM

Despite the fact that New Zealand, like Australia, exhibits 'very conformist medical establishments' (Dew, 2003:30), many New Zealand general practitioners have over the past few decades come to express a strong interest in complementary medicine. As early as some 20 years ago, New Zealand biomedical physicians, particularly general practitioners, were both referring their patients to CAM practitioners and even utilising CAM therapies. A survey of 173 general practitioners in Wellington, the national capital, found that 27 percent of them were practising at least one CAM therapy (Hadley, 1988). A slightly later survey of 249 doctors in Auckland revealed that of 249 respondents in a survey sent to about 700 Auckland biomedical physicians, 171 (68.7 percent) of them referred patients for one or more

CAM treatments and 75 (30 percent) actually practiced one or more CAM therapies (Marshall et al., 1990). The study also found that

> [F]emale doctors tended to refer more, 35 out of 43 (81.4%) compared with 136 out of 206 (665) males ($p = 0.048$). Younger doctors referred to alternative medicine more than older ones, the mean age of referring doctors being 41.2 against 48.6 for those not referring ($p < 0.001$)(Marshall, 1990:214).

A recent survey found that 20 percent of GP respondents practiced one or more CAH therapies and 95 percent referred patients to CAH practitioners (Poynton, Dowell, Dew, & Egan, 2006).

Miskelly (2006), in addition to interviewing eight CAM practitioners and nine 'orthodox' biomedical physicians, interviewed six 'Dr-CAMs' or 'integrative practitioners' (biomedical physicians who utilise CAM therapies in their practices). She reports that all of the Dr-CAMs in her study developed an interest early on in their biomedical careers (Miskelly, 2006:174). Furthermore, Miskelly (2006:174) found that '[d]octors who practised metaphysical therapies, such as mind–body and anthroposophical medicine, are less likely to have a formal qualification as opposed to doctors who use modalities such as acupuncture, manipulation or homoeopathy and naturopathy'. The Dr-CAM's asserted that their integration of CAM therapies into their general practice broadened their scope of practice in order to meet patient demand (Miskelly, 2006:217).

New Zealand nurses have also become interested in incorporating CAM therapies into their treatment regimens as evidenced by frequent references to it in nursing publications (Dew & Kirkman, 2002:145). Maddocks (1995) argues that nurses may find massage and aromatherapy useful in treating patients.

Sociologist Kevin Dew argues that the boundaries between biomedicine and acupuncture have become illusive in that the latter has come to be practised by not only Chinese medicine practitioners but also biomedical physicians belonging to the New Zealand Medical Acupuncture Society (est. 1981) and physiotherapists. He maintains that the existence of biomedical acupuncturists has served as a major barrier in the efforts of the Chinese medicine practitioners to obtain statutory registration. Although the New Zealand Medical Acupuncture Society became an affiliate of the New Zealand Medical Association (NZMA), at least one biomedical acupuncturist, Mat Tizard (who used a form of electro-acupuncture in diagnosing chemical poisoning), was expelled from the medical register in 1992, fined $NZ1,000, and ordered to pay $NZ157,000 in course costs, although these were reduced by the High Court to $100,000, exclusive of General

Sales Tax. In contrast to competent biomedical physicians who tend to be treated relatively leniently for their transgressions, Tizard, a biomedical heretic, provoked outrage by claiming to have found a treatment for a serious health problem that his colleagues could not easily diagnose or treat. Although complementary therapists have become increasingly popular in New Zealand, Dew argues that the growing emphasis on evidence-based medicine, standardisation of procedures, quality assurance, and measurement threatens to delimit both biomedicine and complementary medicine. Aside of the merits or liabilities associated with evidence-based medicine, the University of Otago's Christchurch School of Medicine and Health Sciences maintains a website on complementary and alternative medicine (www.otago.ac.nz, accessed 29/06/2007) that reflects the predilection of biomedicine to subject CAM therapies to this approach.

Summary

As in Australia, complementary medicine has undergone processes of both popularisation and legitimation in New Zealand. Chiropractic and osteopathy more or less function as fully professionalised heterodox medical systems in New Zealand in terms of enjoying statutory registration. However, unlike Australia where all chiropractic training programs are situated in public universities, the sole chiropractic school in New Zealand is a private one. Ironically, osteopathy, a smaller profession, has its training program situated in a public tertiary institution. Other complementary medical systems, such as naturopathy, Western herbalism, and Chinese medicine, lack statutory registration in New Zealand. Furthermore, training programs in these complementary systems are situated entirely in private schools. Like in Australia, a growing number of biomedical physicians and nurses in New Zealand have been incorporating complementary therapies into their practices.

Chapter 9

Government interest in complementary and alternative medicine

Introduction

Despite the fact that Australia and New Zealand have medical systems that are dominated by biomedicine, other medical systems, as this book demonstrates, persist and even thrive, albeit often under precarious or tentative conditions. Indeed, biomedicine's dominance over rival medical systems has never been absolute in any society, developed or developing. In advanced capitalist societies, the state, which primarily serves the interests of the corporate class, must periodically make concessions to subordinate social groups in the interests of maintaining social order and the capitalist mode of production. As a result, certain heterodox or alternative practitioners, with the backing of clients and particularly influential patrons, were able to obtain legitimation in the form of at least limited practice rights and in the cases of osteopathic medicine full practice rights in the United States and homoeopathy in Great Britain.

The Australian scenario

As in other developed societies, the corporate class and the state in Australia since the 1970s have come to express concern about rising health costs. Factors that contributed to rising health costs in Australia, particularly prior to the 1990s, have included (1) an increase in the utilisation of health services, (2) an ageing population, (3) the growth in capital-intensive biotechnology, (4) mismanagement in health care delivery, (5) a capital-intensive provider-driven health care system, and (6) an increase in pharmaceutical expenditures (Hancock, 2002:66). Najman reports,

> Between 1984–85 and 1993–94, the average number of Medicare services per person increased from 7.2 to 10.2. This increase has steadily continued until 2000–01, when there were eleven Medicare services per capita per year for the Australian population. These services are divided in the following way: five unreferred services to general practitioners, emergency and related services; slightly over three pathology

services per person per year; and one specialist service per person per year (Najman, 2003:549).

Between 1989–90 and 1999–2000, health care costs rose from 7.5 percent to 8.5 percent of the Australian GDP (Najman, 2003:530).

In order to address rising health costs, the Australian government has relied upon several strategies: (1) covert rationing that entails limiting public health funds for particular patients or services, such as withdrawal of Viagra on the Pharmaceutical Benefits Scheme; (2) the allocation of patients awaiting surgery to a priority level; (3) increased co-payments for physician visits necessitated by practices such as physicians refusing to bulk bill because they feel that Medicare does not compensate them adequately for services rendered; and (4) the 'establishment of an independent regulator for the private health insurance industry, with responsibility for overseeing premium setting, solvency rules, and takeovers' (Podger & Hagan, 2000:128). However, it is rarely mentioned in the health economics literature that the growing support in various ways for complementary medicine exhibited by the Australian government may constitute another covert strategy for curtailing rising health costs. Indeed, one perspective on the growing popularity of alternative or complementary medicine in developed countries is summarised by Siahpush as follows,

> The enormous amount of money that flows out of the capitalist class (e.g, in the form of workers' compensation) and the State (e.g. in the form of national health coverage) into the hands of health professionals and hospitals is a hindrance for capital accumulation. Many corporate sectors now opt for less expensive, less technological and more holistic modes of healing. Consequently, individuals are encouraged to take the responsibility for their health into their own hands and opt for non-technological and inexpensive therapies (Siahpush, 1999:163).

Given that complementary medical systems, such as naturopathy, homoeopathy, and Chinese medicine, often emphasise individual responsibility for health, they are compatible with the strong interest among government health administrators, health policy makers, and academics in preventive medicine and health promotion. Since the 1970s, both Labor and Coalition governments have encouraged citizens to obtain private health insurance and have sought to make them more self-reliant and responsible (Krieken et al., 2000:159; White, 2002:95). According to Fullagar (2002:70), governmental power in Australia has been 'exercised through a form of rationality (particular truths and logics about healthy living) that is implicit in the processes of self-examination, self-care and self-improvement'.

Under the Labor governments of the 1980s and 1990s, as Kapferer (1996:145) observes, deregulation, privatisation, and 'freedom of choice' became 'benchmarks of quality in fields as diverse as **health** [emphasis mine], education and the welfare of the elderly or infirm'. These policies were justified on the grounds that they would make Australia more competitive in the global economy and have been even more forcibly been promoted by the Liberal-National Coalition which governed between 1996 and 2007. According to Wiseman (1998:63), '[t]he Howard Government's first budget in 1996 demonstrated a determination to reduce dramatically Commonwealth involvement in social and community services, ranging across **health and dental services** [emphasis mine], home and community care, migrant support programs, child care, labour-market programs, and university facilities and fees'. Nevertheless, the Coalition was not able to dismantle Medicare because its popularity with the vast majority of the Australian electorate.

According to Gardner and Barraclough,

> Previous overt hostility towards Medicare on the part of the Liberal-National Coalition has mellowed into a grudging acceptance of the scheme as a continuing institution wide popular – and hence electoral – support. In the 2001 Budget, the scope of Medicare was actually enlarged for the first time since its inception by allocating funds to subsidises visits to psychologists (Gardner & Barraclough, 2002:6).

Like other advanced capitalist societies, Australia has a long tradition of state support for private economic interests (Ravenhill, 1993). The upper echelons of Australian government bureaucracies, including health ones, have increasingly been influenced by 'economic rationalism' – the belief that the 'market is the best way of allocating goods and services in society at large, and that state bureaucracies should adopt business-like principles of management' (Petersen, 1994a:97). Economic rationalism 'promotes the use of competition, advocates consumer choice linked to user payments, rejects the use of government provision of services, and would eliminate welfare payments' (Hall & Viney, 2000:51). The government is viewed as an instrument for creating competitive markets, in part by purchasing services.

While economic rationalism received its initial impetus within the Liberal Party when Malcolm Fraser served as Prime Minister, the Hawke and Keating Labor governments (1983–1996) emphasised it, as did Howard's Coalition government (1996–2007). (Bell & Bell, 1993:120–127; Woodward, 2002:424–436). Indeed, Hancock (1999:1) argues that Australia evolved from a 'wage-earners' welfare state' in the 1980s into 'market and neoliberal state' in the 1990s. More recently,

Castles (2001:542) has observed that 'Labor as well as Liberal – have abandoned … key components of welfare Australian-style'. Economic rationalism calls for a shift of national funds from the public to the private sector. Much of the emphasis of both Labor and Liberal governments for economic rationalism derives from pressures from corporate globalisation. As Beresford observes,

> [G]lobalisation has put great pressure on governments to reduce their social expenditures in order to satisfy the demands of international financial markets. These dictate that the major aims of public policy should be low inflation, low taxation, and reduced government spending (Beresford, 2000:91).

In the case of Australia, it has been a force that has strongly impacted the public sector for over two decades. Australian conservative think tanks have also promoted economic rationalism on the part of various governments (Beder, 2002:89). Of the Organization for Economic Cooperation and Development (OECD) nations, percentage-wise Australia is second only to the United States in private-sector health spending. According to the Australian Institute of Health and Welfare (2000), government funding of health varied from 66.7 percent to 70.0 percent during the decade 1989–1999. The private health sector has been seeking to control more and more biomedical technical and clinical endeavours.

Eastwood (2002:223) maintains that the Australian government's openness to complementary medicine 'emphasises consumer choice and empowerment by promoting increasing knowledge, product safety, and proven efficacy through government regulation of industry'. As Petersen (1994a:194) argues, neo-liberal rationality calls for an 'entrepreneurial individual, endowed with freedom and autonomy'. The Australian government has estimated that over 60 percent of Australians utilise complementary medicine and spend some $2 billion (Australian) on complementary medicine, with about two-thirds of this expenditure going to complementary medicines per se and the remaining third to complementary practitioners (Eastwood, 2002:223). Eastwood (2002) maintains that the government regards complementary health care as preventive medicine that particularly addresses chronic and lifestyle diseases and as means for cutting health care costs. The government's support for complementary medicine is an integral part of its neo-liberal effort to divest itself of much health care expenditure as the Australian public will tolerate.

In 1996 Michael Wooldridge, Minister for Health and Family Services, and Senator Bob Woods, Parliamentary Secretary to the MHFSM invited 73 complementary medicine associations to attend an Alternative Medicines Summit at Old Parliament House (*Final Report of the Alternative Medicines*

Summit, 16 October 1996). Some 80 representatives participated in the meeting.

Wooldridge stated at the Alternative Medicines Summit,

> A growing number of Australians use natural or non-traditional treatment in addition, or as an alternative, to conventional medicine. The Coalition [of the Liberal and National parties] supports the right of Australians to have this free choice ... It accepts that governments need to be engaged with the industry to ensure that consumer needs are met, yet balanced with the need to ensure product and therapy safety and efficacy. It declares that practitioners should be free to practice their disciplines, and that patients and consumers have the right to choose them' (quoted in Australian Complementary Health Association, 1996:6).

Jim Arachne (1997:14), an observer at the Summit, noted that the Government had ruled out the availability of Medicare rebates to complementary medicine practitioners and added that '[t]he Minister reminded questioners that psychologists, podiatrists, dentists, and a range of other health professionals also want Medicare funding and there isn't enough money to go around'. Arachne astutely noted that some observers at the Summit had

> wondered if government concern around complementary medicine might not be based on mainly economic grounds rather than concerns for increasing health and well-being. One calculation estimated savings to government over an election period of around $640 million if just 10% of people with non-serious, self-limiting conditions visited a naturopath rather than a doctor (Arache, 1997:14).

Mark Donohoe, a biomedical general practitioner, also views complementary medicine as a possible cost-cutting measure. He argues,

> In the past decade, complementary and alternative medicine (CAM) has begun to take centre stage in the arena of health maintenance and prevention for increasingly informed, educated, wealthy and predominantly female health consumers, and offers the prospects of significant health benefits at a fraction of the cost of orthodox medical care. This provides an unusual opportunity; namely to improve health outcomes while breaking the cycle of escalation of public health care expenditures (Donohoe, 2003:46).

Finally, sociologist Heather Eastwood (2006:235) argues that the Australian government's pattern of encouraging utilisation of complementary medicine 'reflects a consumerist ideology that supports capitalism through a political rhetoric of choice, rights, and empowerment'.

The Government's MedicarePlus package 'proposes an unprecedented rebate for allied and CAM services when delivered to patients managed through the Enhanced Primary program' (Cohen, 2004b:3). It argues that 'using professionals who complement GPs in care – such as with assessment, treatment management, self-management support, and follow-up – improves patient satisfaction, clinical and health status, and use of health services' (Australian Government Department of Health and Ageing, MedicarePlus Update March 2004, www.health.gov.au/medicreplus/, accessed 25/08/2004).

The Democrats, one of the minor parties in Australia, released a statement in April 2004 calling for a fairer budget balance for health, including certain items pertaining to complementary medicine. They proposed a GST-free status for natural supplements where scientific evidence demonstrates that they are as effective as PBS pharmaceuticals, the development of software providing information to general practitioners on the use of complementary services and products, and funding for research and advice to Government on complementary medicine and services (Australian Democrats. A fairer budget balance for health, April 2004, pp. 2–3).

The Australian government maintains a section on its Health Insite website that focuses 'Complementary and Alternative Therapies' which provides viewers with links to information on acupuncture, Chinese traditional medicine, the regulation and control of complementary therapies and medicines, herbal medicine, homeopathy, naturopathy, chiropractic, and complementary therapies for mental health conditions (Complementary and Alternative Therapies as well as therapies for various complications www.healthinsite. gov.au, accessed 10/09/2004).

On 21–22 September 2006 three parties – the New South Wales Office for Science and Medical Research, the National Health and Medical Research Council, and the Centre for Complementary Medicine – sponsored the 'Complementary Medicine: Future Directions Forum' in Sydney. This event gathered 'together researchers, government and industry representatives involved in complementary medicine research, health care provision, regulation and therapeutic production' in order to discuss the complementary medicine industry in Australia (National Health and Medical Research Council et al., 2006:2). In December 2006 the National Health and Medical Research Council (NHMRC) launched a special call for research applications into complementary medicines. According to Warwick Anderson, NHMRC's Chief Executive Officer,

> The aim of this special $5 million initiative is to fund research that
> will contribute to the body of evidence relating to the use of CM in

Australia. The scope of the funding scheme is broad, encompassing proposals for research into a diverse group of health-related substances,
therapies and disciplines (Anderson, 2007:5).

In 2007, the Australian government granted to $4 million for the cre-
ation of a National Institute of Complementary Medicine that is supported by
the New South Wales government and situated at the University of Western
Sydney. The mandate of the new institute is largely to facilitate research on
complementary medicine and to 'facilitate transition of research effort into
practice and policy, including appropriate integration with the mainstream
health system' (www.nicm.edu.au, accessed 5/01/2009).

Periodically the issue of whether the government should reimburse
complementary practitioners for their services arises. A Medicare Benefits
Review committee chaired by Deputy Robyn Layton of the Administrative
Appeals Tribunal recommended in its report to the Minister of Health in
June 1985 that chiropractic and home birth midwifery be included under
Medicare coverage and that 'some chiropractors should be publicly funded
to work on a salaried or sessional basis in public hospitals and community
health centers' (Willis, 1991:65). The Ministry of Health, however, rejected
these recommendations. While the Australian government has been funding
various complementary medicine training programs, particularly chiropractic, osteopathy, naturopathy, Western herbalism, and Traditional Chinese
Medicine in public universities, undoubtedly because of the low-technology
approaches of these medical systems, the operating costs for these training
programs must be considerably less than those for biomedical schools.

To date, chiropractors and osteopaths constitute the only complementary practitioners who are eligible for reimbursement, albeit on a limited basis, from Medicare. Other than Chinese medicine practitioners in
Victoria, they also are the only complementary practitioners who have been
granted statutory registration. In the event that the Australian government
will ever include other complementary practitioner under Medicare, in all
probability it will require them to hold university degrees rather than simply advanced diplomas and diplomas from private colleges or TAFEs. Aside
of the broader issue of health practitioner competency in general, does statutory registration and a university qualification make or not make a complementary practitioner more qualified to practice his or her therapeutic
modality or modalities? For the most part, complementary practitioners in
Australia have generally not been charged with medical negligence or been
subjected to numerous malpractice suits. A notable exception, however, is
the care of Reginald Fenn who prescribed jojoba drops and an electronic
'Mora machine' in the treatment of a long-term male patient's infant. Nine

days after birth, the infant had been biomedically diagnosed to have a critical aortic stenosis, a condition that requires surgery. Fenn reportedly instructed the parents to 'not let surgeons touch [the infant] because he was too young and would not cope', thus prompting them to cancel a hospital evaluation appointment (quoted in Williams, 2004). With biomedical intervention, the appointment was rescheduled but the infant died before the operation occurred. According to Kerridge, Lowe, and McPhee,

> Mr Fenn pleaded not guilty when he was charged with manslaughter of the 18-day-old baby. The charges were that he was grossly negligent by treating the baby when the problem was beyond his area of expertise. He was sentenced to five years' jail, although the sentence was suspended because he was too ill to serve his time in prison (Kerridge, Lowe, & McPhee, 2005:517).

While it is not clear what kind of naturopathic qualifications he had, the fact that complementary practitioners can practice under Common Law with no formal training or with advanced diplomas or diplomas as opposed to university degrees raises legal and ethical issues beyond the scope of this book.

At any rate, over the last several decades, the status of biomedicine with the context of the Australian dominative medical system has declined due to the growing corporatisation of health care as well as the increasing willingness of the Australian state and its various jurisdictions to give public recognition to complementary medicine. Whereas about 80 percent of biomedical physicians in the early 1970s belonged to the Australian Medical Association, this figure declined to around 50 percent during the 1980s (Petersen, 1994a:87). Various other biomedical associations, particularly the General Practitioners Society in Australia, the Royal Australasian specialty colleges, the Australian Association of Surgeons, and the Doctors' Reform Society had made inroads into its membership.

Collyer (2004) argues that the mainstreaming of complementary medicine is contributing to its co-optation rather than serving to undermine biomedical hegemony. Despite her enthusiasm for complementary medicine, Jill Teschendorff (2001:47), an Associate Professor of Nursing at Victoria University in Melbourne and massage therapist, however, expressed a cautionary note in her assertion that 'holistic medicine' tends to downplay the 'factors in Australian society that jeopardise the health of many Australians', namely those 'related to structural and social organization: to economic rationalism, globalisation, consumerism, and the veneration for individualism'. Indeed, in reality, whatever may have existed of a holistic health movement in Australia has been transformed into complementary medicine or integrative medicine. This process is by no means unique to Australia but also appears to have been occurring in the United States, United Kingdom, and probably in other countries (Baer, 2004).

Stephen Myers (2003), the Director of the Australian Centre for Complementary Medicine, is one of the foremost voices calling for an 'integrated medicine' in Australia – one that draws upon evidence-based medicine and involves collaboration between biomedical practitioners and complementary practitioners. The Australian Centre of Complementary Medicine offers a Graduate Certificate in Evidence-based Complementary Medicine through distance learning for 'doctors, nurses, pharmacists and suitably qualified health professionals who want to improve their knowledge and understanding of evidence-based complementary medicine and how to apply this in their professional practice' (University of Queensland News Online, 2003:1). The Centre has also organised an online conference series on 'Complementary Medicine and Health Education' designed for 'health educators, students and practitioners from orthodox and complementary health backgrounds' (www.accmer.edu.au/conference.htm, p. 1, accessed 24/01/2005).

Peter Sherwood (2005:322) calls for a Voluntary Integrated Model within which the government would fund complementary medicine education, research, and practice: 'In Australia, this would require that free access to the public health system, including hospitals, be extended to natural medicine practitioners and their clients, and that Medicare subsidies for biomedical practices be extended to natural medicine practices'. He asserts, however, that such an arrangement would be acceptable to the cost-conscious Australian governments 'only if they had conclusive proof that there would be a corresponding decrease in biomedicine services and costs, thus rendering the natural medicine funding costs close to budget-neutral' (Sherwood, 2005:323). In contrast to Myers who views evidence-based research as a means for legitimising complementary medicine, Sherwood believes that such an approach would make it less holistic (Sherwood, 2005:334).

In contrast to complementary practitioners who are pushing for statutory registration or the proponents of integrative medicine, Malcolm Parker (2003:1) warns that complementary practitioners are in danger of losing their claim to offering 'truly alternative modalities of healing' if their practices come under increasing governmental regulation. He indicates that the growing emphasis on biomedical-oriented evidence-based efficacy studies of complementary therapies may contribute to the future development of the 'two-tiered structure' under which registered natural products have passed certain efficacy standards and listed ones have been assessed for safety and quality but not efficacy (Parker, 2003:3). Willis and

White (2004:56) contend that while randomised controlled trials associated with evidence-based medicine may lend themselves well where treatment is relatively straightforward, such as in the administration of specific herbal medicines, they observe such an approach becomes much more problematic for complementary medicine because most of treatments entail a 'combination of treatments tailored to individual patients'. Conversely, herbal treatments often involve a combination of herbal substances that are 'tailored to the specific needs of the individual patient' (Wohlmuth, 2003:206). At any rate, the Australian government has been somewhat ambivalent thus far in strictly insisting upon the application of randomised controlled trials (RCTs) to complementary therapies in that it did not call for them when it chose to support the Complementary Therapies Funding Program in February 2002 (Willis & White, 2004:56).

While indeed complementary practitioners, particularly chiropractors and osteopaths, have improved their legitimacy considerably within the context of the Australian dominative medical system, this development has not seriously eroded biomedical domination. As Willis (1988:176) observes, 'Practitioners of complementary care modalities have been so far unsuccessful in gaining access to the hospital system, either public or private'. He further argues that 'medical dominance has changed its form and become more subtle and indirect than previously' (Willis, 1988:179). Conversely, biomedical dominance in Australia overall has been eroding as the federal government and state governments as well as corporations have come to play a more predominant role in the creation of health policy, which in turn have begun to adopt a greater tolerance for complementary medical systems. This growing tolerance, however, is probably more related to the perception that they are cheaper forms of health care than to the fact that they offer competing philosophies of health.

The New Zealand scenario: governmental interest in and support for CAM

Economic rationalism with respect to health care began to appear in New Zealand about the same time that it did in Australia, namely in the 1980s during which time New Zealand developed a 'mixed health economy' (Hindle & Perkins, 2000:93). During this time, the Business Roundtable came to exert a strong influence on health policy reform (Blank, 1994:52). In 1993 the National Party introduced extensive health care reforms which sought to 'introduce competition in the health sector' and encouraged private health service providers to 'compete for contracts with the public health sector to encourage market mechanisms so that health services could be delivered in a fair and efficient manner' (Dew & Kirkman, 2002:88). In a similar vein, Miskelly (2006:iii) argues that the New Zealand state, even under a Labor government, has expressed a strong interest in CAM because its emphasis on patient self-responsibility is consistent with 'neo-liberal and individual-istic discourses'. She argues that a 'neo-liberal climate, with its focus on the role of individuals', provided nurses and CAM providers with an opportu-nity to challenge biomedical dominance (Miskelly, 2006:156).

In 1986, the Department of Health commissioned a report on CAM therapies in New Zealand.

One way that the New Zealand state has given support to CAM with minimal costs has been through recognition on the part of the New Zealand Qualifications Authority of a wide diversity of training programs in a wide array of CAM systems, including naturopathy, aromatherapy, reflexology, remedial body therapies, homeopathy, acupuncture and Chinese medicine (www.newhealth.govt.nz/maccah/training.htm, accessed 03/05/2007). These programs range from weekend workshops and distance-learning courses to four-year, full-time diploma courses.

The Ministerial Advisory Committee on Complementary and Alternative Health (MACCAH) was created in June 2001 under section 11 of the New Zealand Public Health and Disability Act, 2000 (www.newhealth.govt.nz/maccah, accessed 03/05/2007). It recognises a public demand to incorporate CAH into the larger New Zealand health care system. The Committee advised the Minister of Health on policies related to CAH, particularly with respect to regulation, consumer information, research, and incorporation of CAH into the larger New Zealand health care system. Its role ended with delivery of a report in June 2004 (Ministerial Advisory Committee on Complementary and Alternative Health, 2004). MACCH adopted the typology of CAM systems and therapies utilised by the National Institute of Health's National Center for Complementary and Alternative Medicine in the United States. This typology recognises the following categories of CAM systems or therapies:

- Group 1: Alternative medical systems which exhibit 'theory and practice that evolved independently of, and often prior to, the biomedical approach' (Ministerial Advisory Committee on Complementary and Alternative Health, 2004:66). Examples of such systems include Ayurveda, Traditional Chinese Medicine, Pacific traditional healing systems, homoeopathy, and naturopathy.
- Group 2: Mind/body/spirit interventions such as hypnotherapy, rebirth-ing, and spiritual healing.
- Group 3: Biological-based therapies such as herbal medicine, homeobo-tanical therapy, and biological therapies.

- Group 4: Manipulative and body-based therapies such as chiropractic, osteopathy, massage, and Alexander technique.
- Group 5: Energy therapies such as Chi kung, Reiki, touch for health, and bioelectromagnetic-based therapies.

MACCAH recommended that practitioners engaged in 'high-risk CAM modalities' should be regulated under governmental legislation and those engaged in 'lower-risk CAM modalities' should self-regulate themselves under their respective professional associations (MACCAH, 2004:5). It recommended that CAH practitioners utilising high-risk modalities should fall under the guidelines of the Health Practitioners Competence Assurance Act, 2003. MACCAH also recommended that both biomedical and CAM training programs include elements of CAM and biomedicine in each other's curriculum and movement toward integration of biomedicine and CAM both in terms of practice and research.

The Accident Compensation Corporation subsidises acupuncture, chiropractic, and osteopathic services provided by designated practitioners.

The Ministry of Health commissioned New Zealand Guidelines to create a website (www.cam.org.nz) on complementary and alternative medicine that indicates four levels of evidence, ranging from 'evidence with a high degree of reliability' to 'some evidence but based on studies without comparable groups' for CAM systems, particularly namely acupuncture, chiropractic, herbal medicine, homeopathy, and osteopathy (www.cam.org.nz, accessed 29/06/2007). The website also provides information on 'other' CAM systems, including naturopathy, aromatherapy, kinesiology, hypnotherapy, reflexology, spiritual healing, and yoga.

Summary

Despite efforts on part of heterodox practitioners, such as osteopaths, chiropractors, naturopaths, herbalists, and later proponents of holistic health beginning in the 1970s to develop alternatives to biomedicine, what in reality has been developing in both Australia and New Zealand is the beginnings of the co-option of complementary medicine in the case of Australia and complementary and alternative health in New Zealand under the rubric of integrative medicine or integrative health care. As Cant and Sharma (1999:432–433) maintain, 'biomedicine is still the most powerful single health-care profession and is unlikely to cease to be so: those forms of alternative medicine that have been most successful in terms of gaining greater public recognition and legitimacy are, on the whole, those that have had the approval of a sizable section of the medical profession'. In a similar vein,

Morton and Morton (1996:151) observe that 'the broad scope of practice granted to an MD by their license [statutory registration in the cases of Australia and New Zealand] allows them to take short, consolidated courses on complex systems of alternative medicine [eg, acupuncture] and then immediately offer them to the public'. Increasingly Australasian biomedical physicians are redefining CAM therapies as modalities within biomedicine or at least closely related to biomedicine.

Complementary practitioners vary in the extent which they wish to be either accepted by or integrated with biomedicine. In large part, statutory registration tends to force complementary medical systems to biomedicalise their training programs, treatment regimens, and research, such as in the case of adopting evidence-based medicine. Grace et al. (2007) indirectly provide support for my assertion in their comparison of chiropractic and naturopathic curricula in Australia. In their study, they compared the curricula at three chiropractic training programs, all of which are situated in public universities, and 17 naturopathic training programs, four of them situated in public universities and the remainder in private colleges and TAFEs. They report,

> On average, chiropractic courses allocated 45.9% of their curricula to medical sciences, whereas university-based naturopathy courses allocated 26.2% to medical science and non-university naturopathy courses allocated 23% (Grace et al., 2007:19).

Both in Australia and New Zealand, chiropractic enjoys statutory registration, whereas naturopathy does not in either country. While the chiropractic curricula still include subjects dealing with chiropractic philosophy and techniques, the naturopathic curricula contain more space for CAM subjects, such as naturopathic history and philosophy, Western herbal medicine, nutrition, homeopathy, and massage. Even controversial modalities such as iridology and reflexology are taught in at least some Australasian naturopathic training programs.

Up until mid-2007, the Australian government has provided some limited funding, in the order of $5 million in grant funds through the National Health and Medical Research Council for CAM efficacy (www.health.gov. au). In mid-June 2007, the federal government made a commitment to grant the University of Western Sydney $4 million in order to assist this institution in the establishment of a National Institute for Complementary Medicine (National Institute for Complementary Medicine to be established, 19 June 2007, www.health.gov.au). On 30 March, the new Labor government under Prime Minister Kevin Rudd pledged that it would provide over $7 million for research on complementary medicine (Complementary medicine gets a boast, National Health and Medical Research Council, 30 March 2008, www. nhmrc.gov.au). A grant of $1.74 million has been designated for the establishment of three National Institute of Complementary Medicine (NICM) Collaborative Centres to be situated at the University of Queensland, the University of Sydney, and Swinburne University of Technology and another $5.3 million for 13 projects. Senator Jan McLucas, the Parliamentary Secretary to the Minister of Health and Ageing, predicted that the three centres would attract an additional $7.5 million in grants from universities and research funding. Ironically, none of the Collaborative Centres will be situated in a complementary medicine training institution.

Biomedicine historically has often incorporated alternative medicine rather than losing patients en mass to heterodox practitioners. Cross-cultural research has repeatedly indicated that that integration of biomedicine and CAM tends to preserve rather than eradicate biomedical dominance (Baer, 2004; Fadlon, 2005; Saks, 2003). While the development of integrative medicine has not progressed as far in Australia and New Zealand as it has in North America and the United Kingdom, there are strong indications that biomedicine, often with state support, maintained its dominance over complementary, and alternative medicine in Australasia.

On the surface, the holistic health movement, CAM, and even integrative medicine, albeit in descending order, appear to be more *holistic* than biomedicine in that they all posit body–mind–spirit connections. Conversely, all three tend to adopt an individualistic perspective that is compatible with capitalist ideology in that they emphasise internal personal changes rather than external social structural changes.

At any rate, in a matter of a few decades, it appears that biomedicine, governments, and various corporate entities, not only in North America and the United Kingdom but also in Australasia, have domesticated holistic health as a popular movement and transformed it initially into CAM and more recently integrative medicine, a system in which certain complementary or alternative therapies function as adjuncts to high-tech biomedicine. Ian Coulter and I recently co-edited a special issue of *Health Sociology Review* which explores the relationship between biomedicine and complementary and alternative medicine under the guise of integrative medicine in Canada, the United States, the United Kingdom, Australia, and New Zealand (Baer & Coulter, 2008a, 2008b). This transformation constitutes yet one more example of the ability of corporate capitalism and its political allies to co-opt counter-hegemonic movements around the globe. Unfortunately CAM therapists, including those in Australia and New Zealand, often have been inadvertently complicit in this process of domestication.

Chapter 10

Conclusion – How holistic is complementary medicine?

*P*roponents of complementary and alternative medicine and integrative medicine have all too often treated the notion of holistic health as a rhetorical device that serves their own ends, including professional and pecuniary ones, rather than as a substantive one that provides a critique of the existing capitalist world system, its role in contributing to disease, and nationally based dominative medical systems. For the most part, most proponents of holistic health as well as many CAM practitioners and holistically oriented biomedical practitioners tend to a subscribe to a limited holism that emphasises mind–body–spirit connections but generally leaves the larger social and natural environments out of the equation or at best gives them lip service. Like many other alternative medical systems that claim to be holistic, the following characterisation delineated by Cant and Sharma applies to much of what naturopathy in various socio-cultural settings does:

> Holistic health care, radical in some respects, is not at all incompatible with bourgeois notions of individual responsibility, and the new stress on personal growth and energy (not just disease) is in tune with the greater stress on self employment, flexibility of work forces, etc. In turn, alternative medicine like biomedicine distracts attention from the social patterning of illness and offers no attempts to improve the social conditions in which people live. Consequently, there is a sense in which alternative medicine, besides liberating and empowering, actually 'remedicalizes' many areas of life, and it is not difficult to see that there is a consistency between certain capitalist values and the values inherent in many new health practices (Cant & Sharma, 1999).

Despite pressures to coopt complementary and alternative medicine and the notion of holism, there is evidence that a more holistic integrative medical system may eventually emerge in Australasia and elsewhere. As noted earlier, the School of Natural and Complementary Medicine at Southern Cross University developed a Basic Model of (W)holistic Medicine in 1999 which recognises six elements in whole-person care: (1) physical; (2) mental; (3) spiritual; (4) family; (5) community; and (6) environment (Myers et al., 2003:55–56).

While the Southern Cross University model does recognise mind–body–spirit–society connections, it is limited in that it strongly parallels other multi-factorial models of disease etiology in public health and the medical ecological or biocultural perspective in medical anthropology.

More recently, Kim Tippens, a US naturopathic physician and licensed acupuncturist, and her colleague Erin Connelly at the Helfgott Research Institute based at the National College of Natural Medicine in Portland, Oregon, argue that naturopathic medical definitions of holism and wellness,

> should be broadened to address [the] social determinants of health, which falls in line with the naturopathic principal of identifying and treating the underlying causes of illness. To heal the whole person, physicians must take into account that powerful social inequities make it difficult to access and pay for medical care, and can harm one's health (Tippens & Connelly, 2007:783).

Indeed, Tippens and Connelly (2007:783) assert that naturopathic physicians, along with other complementary and alternative medicine practitioners, have a 'a valuable role to play in public health and are in an ideal position to practice "pro-poor" health care, due to their holistic orientation toward health and emphasis on preventive care'.

Given the still small size of complementary and alternative medicine around the world, progressive CAM therapists and biomedical physicians need to become part and parcel of a larger process of advocating an authentically holistic health paradigm which recognises that health and disease are ultimately embedded in political, economic, social structural, and ecological processes (Baer et al., 2003). Howard Waitzkin (2000:204), a critical sociologist and progressive biomedical physician, argues that '[b]ecause of the powerful economic and political interests that dominate the health-care system, the alternative [or holistic] movement cannot succeed unless it connects itself to broader political activism as well'. In the US context, the creation of a universal health care system could pave the way to provide CAM therapies, including naturopathic care, to working class and poor people. Indeed, Waitzkin (2000:205) asserts that '[c]omponents of alternative medicine [may] ultimately also be useful in low-income and minority communities'. In the case of countries with nationalised health care, such as Canada, Britain, Australia, and New Zealand, naturopathic and other CAM therapies could be incorporated into an integrative health system in which biomedical and CAM practitioners work as equals in a collaborative relationship that blends an emphasis on both preventive and curative care.

An authentically holistic and pluralistic medical system would not simply extend access of CAM, including folk medical systems, to working class, peasants, and Indigenous peoples but would need to be part and parcel of global social transformation that would provide all with the benefits of both biomedicine and heterodox healing systems. Ultimately, this assertion applies to Australia and New Zealand as well as all developed and developing societies.

The future of complementary medicine, as well as integrative medicine, in both Australia and New Zealand is difficult to predict but will be subject to numerous larger political, economic, and social structural forces in both societies. So long as complementary medicine by-and-large is not incorporated into the national health plans of Australia and New Zealand, they will tend to continue to serve primarily the more affluent sectors of the two countries. As health sociologist John Gray (2006:245) observes, patients who utilise complementary medicine 'represent a generally more privileged segment of the Australian population'. Undoubtedly the same observation applies for patients who utilise complementary and alternative medicine in New Zealand. Furthermore, although chiropractors, osteopaths, naturopaths, Western medicine practitioners, homeopaths, and Chinese medicine practitioners view themselves as primary care practitioners, as long as they cannot practice in hospitals on a regular basis, they will remain subordinate partners in the dominative medical systems of Australia and New Zealand.

APPENDIX

Appendix 1 – Selected listing of CM journals in Australia

The Art of Healing – Byron Bay (popular)
Australasian Chiropractic and Osteopathy
Australasian Health & Healing: Journal of Alternative Medicine (popular)
Australian Chiropractor Magazine
Australian Journal of Medical Herbalism
Chiropractic and Osteopathic College of Australasia Newsletter
Chiropractic Journal of Australia
Directions: The Journal of Natural Health Professionals.
Diversity – Natural & Complementary Health (Magazine of the Australian Complementary Health Association)(www.diversity.org.au)
Health and Healing: A Holistic Approach to Alternative Living (popular)
Journal of the Australian Traditional-Medicine Society
Journal of Complementary Medicine
Journal of Osteopathic Medicine
The Magnet: Magazine for Spiritual and Complementary Medicine (popular)
Massage Australia
Natural Therapist (official journal of the ANTA)
Review of Traditional Chinese Medicine
Spirit of the Earth Magazine (popular, 1999–2000, covered both complementary and alternative therapies, including New Age healing)

Appendix 2 – Selected listing of complementary medicine associations in Australia

Complementary medicine

Australian Complementary Health Association (est. 1993)(www.diversity.org.au)
Australian Comprehensive Medicine Association

Naturopathic and natural therapies

Alumni Association of Natural Medicine Practitioners: Consists of counsellors, herbalists, homoeopaths, and naturopaths (www.alumni.org.au).
Australian Committee of Natural Therapies (est. 1990)(www.acont.org.au).

Australian Naturopathic Network (est. 1998): Functions as a loose clearing-house for selected complementary medicine associations (www.ann.com.au).

Australian Natural Therapists Association (est. 1955)(www.anta.com.au)

Australian Naturopathic Practitioners Association (est. 1975): Claims to be 'longest standing association of Naturopathy in Australia' and publishes a journal. Its website lists 16 health funds that recognise its members for rebates.

Australasian Federation of Natural Therapists (est. 1996): Was organised by a group of practitioners in Western Australia and now claims over 450 members in Australia and New Zealand.

Academy of Human Sciences: Located in Faliford NSW; offers courses in traditional magic, clinical psychology, and hypnotherapy (www.human-sciences.net.au).

Australian Correspondence Schools: Located in Nerang MDC QLD; offers courses in medicinal aromatherapy, nutrition, life coaching, psychology, well-being and self-sufficiency, and organic farming (www.acs.edu.au).

Brandon Raynor's School of Natural Therapies (est. 2002): Was established by Brandon Raynor, who holds diplomas in naturopathy, remedial massage, shiatsu, Chinese herbalism, Ayurvedic medicine and who has served as the President of the Complementary Medicine Association (est. 1986): Claims to represent 'qualified' complementary practitioners and seeks to educate public as to what naturopaths do, to unite naturopaths in Australia, and to attain full registration for naturopaths in all states (Aims of the CMA, www.cma.asn.au/aims.htm).

Federation of Natural & Traditional Therapists (est. 1991): Consists of various complementary medicine associations and claims to represent the 'great majority of natural and traditional therapists in Australia' and seeks to work with the government and other organisations in order to professionalise complementary medicine (www.fntt.org.au/aboutus.htm, p. 1).

International Natural Therapists Association (www.therapeutic-massage-school.com).

Naturopathic Physician Association of Australia (est. 1972)

Society of Natural Therapists and Researchers (est. 1990)

Whole Health Institute: An educational organization.networking health practitioners and lay people who 'value caring for the whole person and bringing heart into health' (www.wholehealthaustralia.com).

Chinese medicine and acupuncture associations

Acupuncture Association of Australia

Acupuncture Association of Victoria

Aust-China Acupuncture & Chinese Medicine Association
Australian Acupuncture Associated Ltd/Acupuncture Ethics and Standards
 Organisation
Australian Chinese Medical Association (Victoria)
Federation of Chinese Medicine and Acupuncture Societies of Australia
NSW Association of Chinese Medicine
Register of Acupuncture and Traditional Chinese Medicine
Traditional Medicine of China Society Australia
Victorian Traditional Acupuncture Society/Chinese Medicine Association

Osteopathy

Australian Osteopathic Association

Chiropractic

Chiropractors' Association of Australia

Homeopathy

Australian Association of Professional Homoeopaths (www.homoeopathy.
 org.au)
Australian Homeopathic Association (www.homeopathyoz.org)

Australian bush flowers

Australian Bush Flower Essences: Based in Terry Hills NSW (www.ausflow-
 ers.com.au).

Bodywork associations

Association of Remedial Masseurs (www.remedialmasseurs.com.au)
Australian Society of Teachers of the Alexander Technique
 (www.alexandertechnique.org.au)
Australian Pilates Methods Association (www.australian.pilates.asn.au)
Australian Institute of Yoga (www.australian-institute-yoga.com.au)
Felderkrais Guild (www.feldenkrais.org.au)
Infant Massage (www.infantmassage.org.au)
National Council of Massage and Allied Health Practitioners
Pilates Institute of Australasia (North Sydney, www.pilates.com.au): Note:
 Pilates is a system of movement that focuses on body alignment, posture,
 and strengthening and lengthening of bodily muscles in same movement.
 It was developed by German-born Joseph Pilates (1880–1968) who

opened studio in New York in 1926 and introduced his therapeutic system in Australia in 1986 (Heinzman, 2004:58–59)

Professional Massage & Remedial Therapy Society

Queensland Association of Massage Therapists

Shiatsu Therapy Association of Australia (www.staa.org.au)

Tai Chi Association of Australia (www.taichiaustralia.com)

Western Australian Association of Masseurs

Miscellaneous associations

Reika Association of Australia (www.reikionline.com.au)

Australian Hypnotherapists' Association (www.ahahypnotherapy.org)

Australian Reiki Connection: Based in Kalorama VIC (www.australianreiki-connection.com.au)

Australian Society of Clinical Hypnotherapy (www.asch.com.au)

Australian Association of Homotoxicology (est. 2002)

International Federation of Aromatherapists

Appendix 3 – Selected listing of private complementary medicine colleges in Australia

Colleges of natural therapies or complementary medicine

Academy of Safe Therapies: Located in Burleigh Junction QLD; sponsored but independent of SAFE group of companies; offers the Advanced Diploma of Naturopathy and Advanced Diploma and the Diploma of Western Herbalism (www.safetherapies.com.au).

Adelaide Training College of Complementary Medicine: Offers Advanced Diplomas in Acupuncture and Herbal Medicine and also offers programs of study in nutrition and qi gong (www.naturaltherapiescollege.com).

Australian Institute of Applied Sciences: Offers through on-campus and distance education the Bachelor of Naturopathy, Advanced Diploma of Naturopathy, the Advanced Diploma of Applied Science (Acupuncture), the Advanced Diploma of Homeopathy, the Advanced Diploma of Western Herbal Medicine, and other forms of certification. Located in Stones Corner OLD (www.aias.com.au).

Australian Institute of Holistic Medicine: Administered by biomedical practitioners and offers Advanced Diplomas in Naturopathy (Natural Medicine), Western Herbal Medicine, Homoeopathy, Ayurveda; the Diploma of Massage; Graduate Diplomas of Naturopathy, Western Herbal Medicine, Homeopathy, Ayurveda, and Clinical Acupuncture;

the Certificate IV in Massage); its Advanced Diploma in Naturopathy can be articulated for degree status through the University of New England (www.aihm.wa.edu.au/entry.html).

College of Nepean Natural Therapeutics (est. 1980): Offers courses in various natural therapies at the diploma and certificate levels (www.natural-college.com).

Endeavour College of Natural Health: Fuller description in text of book (www.acnm.edu.au)

Gracegrove College: Offers the Advanced Diploma of Medical Herbalism which can lead to the Bachelor of Health Science (Herbal Medicine) through a partnership with Charles Sturt University; also offers the Advanced Diploma in Remedial Message that can lead to Bachelor of Health Science (Remedial Massage) again through a partnership with Charles Sturt University; also offers the Advanced Diploma of Psychotherapy and the Diploma of Esoteric Sciences and Holistic Counselling, the Diploma of Dream Therapy, Interpretation & Analysis, and the Certificate IV in Massage. Esoteric Sciences focuses upon existential issues and incorporates Zen philosophy, mystic powers of music, psychology of flower essences, goddess within, meditation, numerology, astrology, rays, etc. (www.gravegrovecolleges.net).

Hannya Medical College of Naturopathic & Chinese Medicine: Located in Habersfield, New South Wales (www.hannyamedicalcollege.com).

HealthQuest: Offers online courses at the introductory, diploma, masters, and doctoral levels. Its two-year diploma course is accredited by the International Medicine Ways Institute (www.healthquest.com.au).

Health Schools Australia: Located in Runaway Bay QLD; specialises in distance learning (www.healthaustralia.com).

International College of Complementary Medicine: Started out as New South Wales College of Naturopathic and Osteopathic Medicine in 1967 and became the Health Schools in Australia in 1987 (Martyr: 274). It offers the Advanced Diploma of Complementary Medicine (6 streams), the Diploma of Natural Medicine (6 streams), the Certificate IV in Natural Therapies (4 streams)(www.healthaustralia.com).

Kim Dudley Naturopathy College: Located in Griffth ACT; operates in conjunction with a natural products dispensary and the clinical practitioners of four complementary practitioners; offers a homeopathy certificate, an Ayurveda certificate, short-term classes for the general public, and publishes *The Natural Physician* (www.thehierophant.com.au).

Laws College of Naturopathy (est. 1971): Located in Ringwood VIC. This college was created after some disenchanted Southern School of Natural

Therapies students approached a Mrs Law about starting a rival naturopathic school which initially was called the Laws College of Naturopathy and Chiropractic (Canaway, 2007:50–52).

National College of Traditional Medicine (est. 1987): Located in Sunshine VIC; offers Advanced Diploma in Naturopathy, Certificate IV in Massage, and Diploma in Remedial Massage (www.nctm.com.au).

National Institute of Health Sciences (est. 1995): Located in Deakin West, ACT; offers the Bachelor of Naturopathy, the Advanced Diploma of Naturopathy, and the Advanced Diploma of Acupuncture. (www.nihs. com.au).

Nature Care College: Offers advanced diplomas in naturopathy, *see others*.

NSW School of Natural Medicine: Located in Coffs Harbour NSW; offers the Advanced Diploma of Naturopathy (www.nswsnm.com.au).

Paramount College of Natural Medicine: Offers the Advanced Diploma of Naturopathy (paramounthealth@aol.com).

Perth Academy of Natural Therapies (est. 1988): Offers the Advanced Diploma in Naturopathy, the Advanced Diploma in Traditional Chinese Medicine, and the Diploma in Remedial Massage (www.pant.wa.au).

Robyn Morro's College of Natural Medicine: Offers the Advanced Diploma of Naturopathy, the Advanced Diploma of Western Herbal Medicine, and various Certificate (www.robynmorro.com.au).

South Australian College of Natural and Traditional Medicine (est. 1980): Offers courses in acupuncture, aromatherapy, nutrition, massage, naturopathic sports medicine.

Colleges of acupuncture and Traditional Chinese Medicine

Academy of Traditional Chinese Medicine in Australia
Acupuncture College of Melbourne
College of Traditional Chinese Medicine
Sydney Institute of Traditional Chinese Medicine

Schools of homoeopathy

Academy of Homeopathic Medicine: Located in Highgate Hill QLD; offers the Advanced Diploma of Homeopathy (www.hommedcentre.com).

Australasian College of Hahnemannian Homoeopathy: Located in Daylesford VIC (users.netconnect.com.au)

Sydney College of Homeopathic Medicine, Ashfield, NSW. (www.schm. edu.au)

Schools of massage therapy and other forms of bodywork

All Regions Massage School: Located in Rowville VIC.

Australian College of Sports Therapy: Offers Advanced Diploma in Remedial Massage (Myotherapy) and Diploma of Remedial and Sports Massage. Located in Caulfield, Victoria (www.sportstherapy.edu).

Australian School of Therapeutic Massage: Offers Diploma of Remedial Massage; located in Camberwell, Victoria (www.astm.com.au).

Australian Shiatsu College: Offers Diploma of Shiatsu and Oriental Therapies; Located in Collingwood, Victoria (www.australianshiatsucollege.com.au).

College of Complemetary Medicine: Located in Sydney and Melbourne (www.complementary.com.au).

East West College of Natural Therapies (est. 1978): Formerly Shiatsu Australia; located in South Caulfield, Victoria; Offers Diploma of Remedial Massage, Diploma of Shiatsu and Oriental Therapies; Certificate IV in Massage; and Basic Certificates in Massage and Shiatsu (www.eastwestcollege.com.au).

ESTT College of Natural Medicine: Offers Diploma of Remedial Massage; located in Mulgrave, Victoria (www.estt.vic.edu.au).

Melbourne Institute of Massage Therapy: Offers Diploma of Remedial Massage; located in Heidelberg, Victoria (www.rmit.edu.au/compmed

Moods School of Massage: Located in Dandenong, Victoria.

New School of Therapeutic Massage: Located in Sydney.

Nova School of Massage and Body Therapy: Established Newcastle NSW 1982; Armidale NSW and Lismore NSW 1994.

School of Wholistic Massage: Located in Camberwell, Victoria.

Steve Lockhart's Myotherapy School and Clinic (www.sim-boydwork.com).

Verona Therapy & Beauty Academy: Located in Ashmore, Gold Coast QLD (www.veronaacademy.com.au).

Victorian College of Health Care Education: Offers Advanced Diploma of Myotherapy; located in Moorabbin, Victoria (www.vche.com.au).

White Horse School of Massage & Natural Therapies: Located in Kincumber NSW.

Schools of reflexology

Reflexology Academy of Brisbane: Located in Greenslopes QLD.

West Australian School of Reflexology: Located in Wembley WA.

Australian School of Reflexology (est. 1990): Located in Nords Wharf NSW (www.reflexologyaustralia.com).

Australian College of Chi-Reflexology: Located in Hazelbrook NSW (www.chi-reflexology.com.au).

Miscellaneous schools

Australian College of Health Sciences: Located in Mt. Pleasant WA: Operates the Australian School of Natural Beauty and Spa Therapies and the Australian School of Clinical Aromatherapy.

Australian College of Therapeutic Touch: Based in Hobart, Tasmania.

Australian Foundation for Healing Touch (www.healing.touch.org.au).

Australian School of Clinical Aromatherapy (est. 1994)(www.aroma-therapy. com.au).

School of Aromatic Medicine: Located in Wamberal NSW.

Ayurveda Awareness Centre: Located in Perth; offers the Advanced Diploma of Ayurveda.

Australian School of Awareness: Located in Mooroolbark, Victoria (www. australianschoolofawareness.net).

International House of Reiki: Located in Glebe NSW (www.reiki.net.au).

Essence of Healing: Located in Drouin, Victoria; offers courses on emotions and flower essences.

Australian College of Phytotherapy: Located in Warwick QLD (www.herbaleducation.com.au).

Appendix 4 – Public Universities and TAFEs with complementary medicine training programs

Royal Melbourne Institute of Technology University: Offers Bachelor of Applied Science with streams in Chiropractic and Osteopathy and the Bachelor of Applied Science (Chinese Medicine/Human Biology); Marc Cohen, a biomedical physician with extensive studies in TCM, is the founding head of the Department of Complementary Medicine at RMIT (Cohen, 2003).

Macquarie University: Offers BSc and MSc in Chiropractic (www.chiro. mq.edu.au/chiro/chdpt.htm).

Murdoch University: Located in Perth; offers BSc and MSc in Chiropractic.

Southern Cross University, Department of Natural and Complementary Medicine (est. 1997): Located at Lismore NSW; offers the Bachelor of Naturopathy, the Bachelor of Naturopathy with Honours, the Bachelor of Natural Therapies, the Graduate Certificate in Evidence-based Complementary Medicine, and the PhD in Natural Medicine; probably is the first government-funded university world-wide to order a degree in Naturopathy; Southern Cross University held a conference on 'Herbal Medicine into the New Millennium' in 16–18 June 1999 (Lewis, 1999) (www.scu.edu.au/schools/ncm).

University of Western Sydney – Campbelltown: Offers BSc and MSc in Osteopathy; a three-year Bachelor of Health Sciences (Naturopathy) in conjunction with Endeavour College in Sydney; BSc and MSc in Chinese medicine.

University of New England: Located in Armidale NSW; offers the Master of Health Science (Herbal Medicine) in conjunction with the Australian College of Phytotherapy.

University of Newcastle: Started offering the Bachelor of Natural Therapies in 2002 but dropped this program; has built upon the framework of the Diploma of Medical Herbalism offered through Southern Cross Herbal School, a Division of the University of Newcastle Research Associates (www.newcastle.edu.au).

University of Technology, Sydney: Offers the Bachelor of Science in Traditional Chinese Medicine (www.uts.edu.au).

Victoria University of Technology: Offers MSc in Acupuncture and BSc in Traditional Chinese Medicine; offers Master's Degree in Osteopathy.

Canberra Institute of Technology: Offers the Advanced Diploma of Naturopathy through Department of Health Sciences. Students can study naturopathy on a full-time or a part-time basis at the Bruce campus; those students who wish entry into a university after having completed the Advanced Diploma can apply for credit transfer into a number of degree programs.

Academy of Natural Therapies (TAFE – Gold Coast). Offers Advanced Diplomas in Health Science (Acupuncture), Naturopathy, and Western Herbal Medicine (www.goldcoast.tafe.net).

Brenner Institute of TAFE in Queensland: Offers Advanced Diploma of Naturopathy.

TAFE – Tasmania in Hobart: Offers the Advanced Diploma of Naturopathy (www.tafe.tas.edu.au).

Appendix 5: CAM organisations in New Zealand

Aquatic Bodywork Association of New Zealand
Australasian Chiropractic Society
Healing Touch New Zealand
Hellerwork Association of New Zealand
Homeobotanical Institute
Hypnotherapy Industry Advisory Group
International Research into Iridology and Scerology
Kinesiology Practitioners Accreditation Board
Magnetic Healers Unlimited

Massage Institute
National Federation of Spiritual Healers
Natural Healing Research Institute
Natural Health Council (www.naturalhealthcouncil.org.nz)
Natural Therapies Limited
New Zealand Acupuncture Standards Authority
New Zealand Association of Anthroposophical Doctors
New Zealand Association of Jin Shin Jyutsu
New Zealand Association of Medical Herbalists
New Zealand Association of Professional Hypnotherapists
New Zealand Association of Rebirthers and Breathworkers
New Zealand Bowen Therapy
New Zealand Charter of Health Practitioners
New Zealand Chiropractors Association
New Zealand Council of Homeopaths
New Zealand Feldenkrais Guild
New Zealand Homoeopathic Society (www.homoeopathica.org.nz)
New Zealand Institute of Acupuncture
New Zealand Light and Colour Therapy
New Zealand Natural Health Practitioners Accreditation Board
New Zealand Natural Medicine Association (www.nznma.com)
New Zealand Register of Acupuncturists
New Zealand Registrar of Homeopathics
New Zealand Society of Clinical and Applied Hypnotherapy
New Zealand Therapeutic Laser Association
NZ Society of Naturopaths (www.naturopath.org.nz)
Osteopathic Council of New Zealand (www.osteopathiccouncil.org.nz)
Osteopathic Society of New Zealand (www.osnz.org)
Psychotherapy and Hypnotherapy Institute of New Zealand
Reflexology New Zealand
Registrar of New Zealand Traditional Chinese Medicine Practitioners
Society of Natural Therapists and Researchers
Therapeutic Massage Association
Wellington Group of Reflexology New Zealand

Appendix 6: CAM schools in New Zealand

Aromaflex International Aromatherapy School: Located in Nelson on South
    Island; offers a Diploma in Reflexology (www.aromaflex.co.nz).
Auckland College of Natural Medicine
Australasian College of Herbal Studies

Austra-Soma Society of New Zealand

Canterbury College of Natural Medicine

Christchurch College of Holistic Healing

Holistic School of Reflexology: Located in Christchurch; offers Certificate Course (www.reflexologytraining.co.nz).

International Institute of Reflexology (New Zealand): Located in Auckland; offers Diploma in Reflexology.

Lotus Holistic Centre: Located in Hastings; offers Certificate Course.

Naturopathic College of New Zealand (New Plymouth): Offers domain accreditations in aromatherapy, complementary therapies, homeobotanical therapy, homoeopathy, massage, and reflexology (www.nzqa.govt.nz).

New Zealand College of Chinese Medicine: Located in Christchurch; offers Certificate in Foundation Studies for Traditional Chinese Medicine, Diploma in Acupuncture-Traditional Chinese Medicine, Diploma in Chinese Herbal Medicine, Diploma in Tui Na, and Diploma in Acupuncture (www.communities.com.nz).

New Zealand School of Clinical Hypnotherapy

New Zealand College of Massage: Located in Wellington and Auckland (www.massage.college.co.nz).

Naturopathic College or New Zealand

New Zealand College of Homeopathy

New Zealand School of Acupuncture and TCM: Has an Auckland Campus and a Wellington Campus (www.chinesemedicine.ac.nz).

Palmerston North School of Reflexology: Offers Certificate Course.

Taranaki School of Massage

Wellington College of Homoeopathy

Wellington School of Massage

Wellpark College of Natural Therapies: Located in Auckland; offers Diploma of Naturopathy, Diploma in Herbal Medicine and Nutrition, Diploma of Ayurvedic Medicine, and Diploma of Maori Healing (www.wellpark. co.nz).

Whitecliffe College of Art and Design

BIBLIOGRAPHY

Abraham, J. (1995). *Science, politics, and the pharmaceutical industry: Controversy and bias in drug regulation.* New York: St. Martin's Press.

Acupuncture Association of Australia. (2000). *A brief history of the Acupuncture Association of Australia 1972–2000.* Belrose, NSW: Acupuncture Association of Australia.

Adams, J., Sibbritt, D. W., Easthope, G., & Young, A. F. (2003). The profile of women who consult alternative health practitioners in Australia. *Medical Journal of Australia, 179*(6), 297–300.

Albrecht, G. L., & Levy, J. A. (1982). The professionalization in osteopathy: Adaptation in the medical marketplace. In J. A. Roth (Ed.), *Research in the sociology of health care, volume 2: Changing structure of health service occupations* (pp. 161–206). Greenwich, CT: JAI Press.

Anderson, W. P. (2007, May/June). Building an evidence base for complementary medicine. *Complementary Medicine,* p. 7.

Andrews, G. J., & Phillips, D. R. (2005). Petit bourgeois health care? The big small-business of private complementary medical practice. *Complementary Therapies in Clinical Practice, 11,* 87–104.

Arachne, J. (1997). Alternative medicines summit: A consumer's view. *Diversity, 1*(10), 13–14.

Australian Acupuncture and Chinese Medicine Association. (2001). *Australian guidelines for traditional Chinese medicine education.* West End, QLD: Australian Acupuncture and Chinese Medicine Association.

Australian Bureau of Statistics. (1983). *National health survey.* Canberra, ACT: Australian Government.

Australian Bureau of Statistics. (1997–1998). *Chiropractic and osteopathic services Australia.* Canberra, ACT: Australian Government.

Australian Bureau of Statistics. (2008). *Australian social trends, 2008,* from http://www.abs.gov.au.

Australian Chiropractors Association (Victorian Branch). (1961). One group for all Australia. *Chiropractic, 3*(3), 5, 8.

Australian Chiropractors Association (Victorian Branch). (1965). ACA directory. *Chiropractic, 4*(1), 28–31.

Australian College of Holistic Nurses. (2000). *Policy guidelines for practice of complementary medicine by nurses and midwives in Australia, November 2000.* Brendale, QLD: Duo Publishers.

Australian College of Natural Medicine. (2006). *Course guide 2006.* Brisbane, QLD: ACNM.

Australian Complementary Health Association. (1996). Alternative medicines summit – Health minister supports alternatives. *Diversity, 1*(9), 6.

Australian Complementary Health Association. (2002). GST drives national proposals for professional registration. *Diversity*, *2*(7), 10.

Australian Institute of Health and Welfare. (2000). *Australia's health service expenditure to 1998/99* (Health Expenditure Bulletin, No. 16). Canberra, ACT: AIHW.

Australian Medical Association. (1992, September). *Chiropractic in Australia* (pamphlet).

Australian Medical Association. (2002). *AMA position statement on complementary medicine*. Barton, ACT.

Australian National Therapists Association. (2004, September). *Response to the parliamentary secretary to the minister of health and aging on the report of the expert committee on complementary medicines in the Australian health system*. Accessed April 29, 2004, from http://www.anta.com.au.

Australian Traditional Medicine Society. (2005, August). *Submission to the Department of Health discussion paper on the registration of practitioners of Chinese medicine in Western Australia*.

Baer, H. A. (1981). The organization rejuvenation of osteopathy: A reflection of the decline of professional dominance in medicine. *Social Science and Medicine, 15A*, 701–711.

Baer, H. A. (1984a). A comparative view of a heterodox health system: Chiropractic in America and Britain. *Medical Anthropology, 8*, 151–168.

Baer, H. A. (1984b). The drive for professionalization in British osteopathy. *Social Science and Medicine, 19*, 717–725.

Baer, H. A. (1987). Divergence and convergence in two systems of manual medicine: Osteopathy and chiropractic in the United States. *Medical Anthropology Quarterly, 1*, 176–193.

Baer, H. A. (2001). *Biomedicine and alternative healing systems in America: Issues of class, ethnicity, race, and gender*. Madison, WI: University of Wisconsin Press.

Baer, H. A., Singer, M., & Susser, I. (2003). *Medical anthropology and the world system: A critical perspective* (2nd ed.). Westport, CT: Praeger.

Baer, H. A. (2004). *Toward an integrative medicine: Merging alternative therapies with biomedicine*. Walnut Creek, CA: Altamira Press.

Baer, H. A., & Coulter, I. (Eds.). (2008a). Special issue – Integrative, complementary and alternative medicines: Challenges for biomedicine. *Health Sociology Review 17*(4), 329–432.

Baer, H. A., & Coulter, I. (Eds.). (2008b). Introduction – Taking stock of integrative medicine: Broadening biomedicine or co-option of complementary and alternative medicine? *Health Sociology Review, 17*(4), 331–341.

Baer, H. A., Singer, M., & Susser, I. (2003). *Medical anthropology and the world system: A critical perspective*. Westport, CT: Praeger.

Baverstock, P. (1999). Introduction. In S. Fechter, et al. (Eds.), *Herbal medicine into the new millennium conference – Lismore NSW 16–18 June 1999* (p. iii). Lismore, NSW: Southern Cross University.

Beder, S. (2002). *Global spin: The corporate assault on environmentalism* (Rev. ed.). Devon: Green Books.

Beer, S. L. (2005). *Chinese herbal medicine and the hot flush*. PhD thesis, Key Centre for Women's Health, University of Melbourne, Australia.

Begbie, S. D., Zoltan, L. K., & David, R. B. (1996). Patterns of alternative medicine use by cancer patients. *Medical Journal of Australia, 165*, 540.

Belcher, H. (2002). Power, politics, and health care. In J. Germov (Ed.), *Second opinion: An introduction to health sociology* (pp. 257–282). Melbourne: Oxford University Press.

Belgrave, M. (1985). *'Medical men' and 'lady doctors': The making of a New Zealand profession, 1867–1941*. PhD thesis, Victoria University of Wellington, New Zealand.

Bell, P., & Bell, R. (1993). *Implicated: The United States in Australia*. Melbourne: Oxford University Press.

Bennett, J. (2002–2003). Alan Bensoussan pursuing research into Chinese medicine. *Diversity, 2*(8), 33–35.

Bennett, J. (2003–2004). Stephen Myers: Healing the rift between natural and orthodox medicine. *Diversity, 2*(9), 13–15.

Bensoussan, A. (1989). *The vital meridian*. Melbourne: Churchill Livingstone.

Bensoussan, A., & Lewith, G. T. (2004). Complementary medical research in Australia: A strategy for the future. *Medical Journal of Australia, 181*(6), 331–333.

Bensoussan, A., & Myers, S. P. (1996). *Toward a safer choice – The practice of traditional Chinese medicine in Australia*. Melbourne: Department of Human Services.

Bensoussan, A., Myers, S. P., Wu, S. M., & O'Connor, K. (2004). Naturopathic and Western herbal medicine practice in Australia – A workforce survey. *Complementary Therapies in Medicine, 12*, 17–27.

Bentley, P. (2000). Physical therapies. *Diversity, 2*(3), 13–18.

Bentley, P. (2005). Herbalists unite to defeat government attack – The 1925 struggle. *Diversity, 2*(10), 40–47.

Beresford, Q. (2000). *Governments, markets and globalisation: Australian public policy*. St. Leonards, NSW: Allen & Unwin.

Berndt, C. H. (1964). The role of native doctors in Aboriginal Australia. In A. Kiev (Ed.), *Magic, faith and healing* (pp. 264–282). New York: Free Press.

Black, A. W. (1991). Australian Pentecostalism in comparative perspective. In A. W. Black (Ed.), *Religion in Australia: Sociological perspectives* (pp. 106–120). Sydney: Allen & Unwin.

Blackmore, M. C. (n.d.). *Pandemonium: Government health policy and complementary medicines*. Unpublished Paper.

Blank, R. H. (1994). *New Zealand health policy: A comparative study*. Auckland: Auckland University Press.

Bloomfield, R. J. (1983). Naturopathy. In R. H. Bannerman, J. Burton, & C. Wen-Chieh (Eds.), *Traditional medicine and health care coverage: A reader for health administrators and practitioners* (pp. 116–123). Geneva: World Health Organization.

Bolton, S. P. (1986). Making it legal 'down under': The struggle for recognition in Australia. *Chiropractic History, 6,* 11–16.

Bolton, S. P. (1989). The future of chiropractic education in New South Wales: A discussion. *Journal of the Australian Chiropractors' Association, 19*(1), 25–28.

Bombardieri, D., & Easthope, G. (2000). Convergence between orthodox and alternative medicine: A theoretical elaboration and empirical test. *Health, 4,* 479–494.

Bottley, G. (1976). Rural Greeks and illness: An anthropologist's viewpoint. *Medical Journal of Australia, 1*(21), 798–800.

Bouma, G. (2006). *Australian soul: Religion and spirituality in the twenty-first century.* Cambridge: Cambridge University Press.

Bowden, R. (1988). *Self-help osteopathy: Help yourself to health.* Chatswood, NSW: Nature & Health Books.

Brighthope, I. (1994). The therapeutic potential of antioxidants in the prevention of degenerative diseases. *Journal of the Australian College of Nutritional and Environmental Medicine, 13*(1), 15–26.

Brooks, P. M. (2004). Undergraduate teaching of complementary medicine. *Medical Journal of Australia, 181*(5), 275.

Brownie, S. (2005). The development of the US and Australian dietary supplement regulations: What are the implications for product quality? *Complementary Therapies in Medicine, 13,* 191–198.

Campbell, S. A., Dillon, J. L., & Polus, B. I. (1982). Chiropractic in Australia: Its development and legitimation. *Journal of the Australian Chiropractors' Association, 12*(4), 21–30.

Campbell, S. A., Dillon, J. L., & Polus, B. I. (1982). Chiropractic in Australia: Its development and legitimation. *Journal of the Australian Chiropractors' Association, 22*(4), 21–30.

Canaway, R. (2007). The study of the development of the naturopathic profession in Melbourne. Master of Social Health thesis, Centre of Health and Society, University of Melbourne, Melbourne, VIC, Australia.

Cant, S., & Sharma, U. (1999). *A new medical pluralism: Alternative medicine, doctors, patients, and the state.* London: Taylor & Francis.

Carlton, A. L. (2003). *Regulation of the health professions in Victoria: A discussion paper.* Melbourne: Policy and Strategic Projects Division, Victorian Government of Human Services.

Carlton, A. L., & Bensoussan, A. (2002). Regulation of complementary medicine practitioners in Australia: Chinese medicine as a case example. *Complementary Therapies in Medicine, 10,* 20–26.

Casey, M. G., Adams, J., & Sibbritt, D. (2007). An examination of the prescription and dispensing of medicines by Western herbal therapists: A national survey in Australia. *Complementary Therapies in Medicine, 15,* 13–20.

Castles, F. G. (2001). A farewell to Australia's welfare state. *International Journal of Health Services*, *31*, 537–544.

Cawte, J. (1974). *Medicine in the law: Studies in psychiatric anthropology of Australian tribal societies*. Honolulu, HI: University of Hawaii Press.

Clavarino, A., & Yates, P. (1995). Fear, faith or rational choice: Understanding the users of alternative therapies. In G. M. Lupton & J. M. Najman (Eds.), *Sociology of health and illness: Australian readings* (2nd ed., pp. 252–273). Melbourne: MacMillan.

Cohen, M. (Ed.). (2002). *Prescriptions for Holistic Health*. Clayton, VIC: Monash Institute of Health Services Research.

Cohen, M. (Ed.). (2003). *Holistic healthcare in practice*. Melbourne: Australasian Integrative Medical Association.

Cohen, M. (Ed.). (2004a). CAM practitioners and 'regular' doctors: Is integration possible? *Medical Journal of Australia*, *180*(12), 645–646.

Cohen, M. (Ed.). (2004b). *Holistic solutions for sustainable healthcare*. Melbourne: Australasian Integrative Medicine Association.

Cohen, M. H. (2000). *Complementary and alternative medicine: Legal boundaries and regulatory perspectives*. Baltimore: Johns Hopkins University Press.

Cohen, M. M., Penman, S., Pirotta, M., & Da Costa, C. (2005). The integration of complementary therapies in Australian general practice: results of a national survey. *Journal of Alternative and Complementary Medicine*, *11*, 995–1004.

Collyer, F. (2004). The corporatisation and commercialisation of complementary and alternative medicine. In P. Tovey, G. Easthope & J. Adams (Eds.), *The mainstreaming of complementary and alternative medicine: Studies in social context* (pp. 81–99). London: Routledge.

Commission of Inquiry. (1979). *Chiropractic in New Zealand: Report of the commission of inquiry*. Wellington: P.D. Hasselberg Government Printer.

Committee of Inquiry. (1977). *Chiropractic, osteopathy, homoeopathy and naturopathy: Report of committee of inquiry* (Parliamentary Paper No. 102). Canberra, ACT: Acting Commonwealth Government Printer.

Committee on the Health Care Complaints Commission. (2005, November). *Report into traditional Chinese medicine* (Report No. 10/53). Sydney: Parliament of New South Wales.

Connor, L. H. (2004). Relief, risk and renewal: Mixed therapy regimens in an Australian suburb. *Social Science and Medicine*, *59*, 1695–1705.

Coulter, I. D., & Willis, E. M. (2004). The rise and rise of complementary and alternative medicine: A sociological perspective. *Medical Journal of Australia*, *180*(11), 587–589.

Crisp, J., & Taylor, C. (2001). *Potter & Perry's fundamentals of nursing*. Sydney: Harcourt Australia.

Cummings, F. J. (2000). Complementary medicine regulation in Australia. *Current Therapeutics*, *41*, 57–61.

Daffy, P. (1998). Herbal medicines: An industry perspective. *Diversity*, *1*(15), 13–17.

Davis, P. (1981). *Health and health care in New Zealand*. Auckland: Longman Paul.

D'Crus, A., & Wilkinson, J. M. (2005). Reasons for choosing and complying with complementary health care: An in-house study on a Southern Australia clinic. *Journal of Alternative and Complementary Medicine*, *11*, 1107–1112.

Department of Health. (2005, November). *Regulation of practitioners of Chinese medicine in Australia: Discussion paper*. Perth: Government of Western Australia.

Devereaux, E. P. (1998). History of chiropractic from a New South Wales perspective (1969–1982). *Australasian Chiropractic and Osteopathy*, *7*(2), 68–79.

Devereaux, E. P., & Sweaney, J. A. (1981). Joint statement of education. *Chiropractic Australia*, *1*(2), 17.

Dew, K. (2003). *Borderland practices: Regulating alternative therapies in New Zealand*. Dunedin: University of Otago Press.

Dew, K., & Kirkman, A. (2002). *Sociology of health in New Zealand*. South Melbourne: Oxford University Press.

Di Stefano, V. (2006). *Holism and complementary medicine: Origins and principles*. Crows Nest, NSW: Allen & Unwin.

Dixon, C. W., Dodge, M. D., Emery, G. M., & Spears, G. F. S. (1997). Attitudes of the public to medical care: Part 8, 'non-medical' practitioners. *The New Zealand Medical Journal*, *85*(579), 1–3.

Donohoe, M. (2003). The cost of CAM – Against. *Journal of Complementary Medicine*, *2*(1), 46–48.

Drury, N. (1985). *Australian sourcebook of natural health*. Melbourne: Pitman.

Duckett, S. J. (2004). *The Australian health care system* (2nd ed.). South Melbourne: Oxford University Press.

Duke, K. (2005). A century of CAM in New Zealand: A struggle for recognition. *Complementary Therapies in Clinical Practice*, *11*(1), 11–16.

Durie, M. (2001). Mauri Ora: The dynamics of Maori health. Auckland: Oxford University Press.

Dwyer, J. M. (2004). Good medicine and bad medicine: Science to promote the convergence of 'alternative' and orthodox medicine. *Medical Journal of Australia*, *180*(12), 647–648.

Dyason, D. (1988). The medical profession in colonial Victoria, 1834–1901. In R. Macleod & M. Lewis (Eds.), *Disease, medicine, and empire: Perspectives on Western medicine and the experience of European expansion* (pp. 194–216). London: Routledge.

Easthope, G. (1993). The response of orthodox medicine to the challenge of alternative medicine in Australia. *Australian and New Zealand Journal of Sociology*, *29*, 289–301.

Easthope, G. (1999). Alternative medicine. In J. Germov (Ed.), *Second opinion: An introduction to health sociology* (pp. 267–280). Melbourne: Oxford University Press.

Easthope, G. (2004). Complementary medicine and orthodox medicine. In C. Grbich (Ed.), *Health in Australia: Sociological concepts and issues* (3rd ed., pp. 310–333). Frenchs Forest, NSW: Pearson Longman.

Easthope, G. (2005). Alternative medicine. In J. Germov (Ed.), *Second opinion: An introduction to health sociology* (3rd ed., pp. 332–348). South Melbourne: Oxford University Press.

Easthope, G., Beilby, J. J., Gill, G. F., & Tranter, B. K. (1998). Acupuncture in Australian general practice: Practitioner characteristics. *Medical Journal of Australia, 169*, 197–2000.

Easthope, G., Tranter, B., & Gill, G. (2000a). General practitioners' attitudes toward complementary therapies. *Social Science and Medicine, 51*, 1555–1561.

Easthope, G., Tranter, B., & Gill, G. (2000b). Normal medical practice of referring patients for complementary therapies among Australian general practitioners. *Complementary Therapies in Medicine, 8*(4), 226–233.

Eastwood, H. (1997). *General medical practice, alternative medicine and the globalisation of health.* PhD thesis, University of Queensland, Australia.

Eastwood, H. (2000). Why are Australian GPs using alternative medicine? Postmodernisation, consumerism and the shift towards holistic health. *Journal of Sociology, 36*, 133–156.

Eastwood, H. (2002). Globalisation, complementary medicine, and Australian health policy: The role of consumerism. In H. Gardner & S. Barraclough (Eds.), *Health policy in Australia* (2nd ed., pp. 224–245). Melbourne: Oxford University Press.

Ebrall, P. S. (2003). Chiropractic. In T. Robson (Ed.), *An introduction to complementary medicine* (pp. 135–151). Crows Nest, NSW: Allen & Unwin.

Evans, S. (2000a). Social change and alternative medicine: A herbalist's view. *Diversity, 2*(1), 17–22.

Evans, S. (2000b). The story of naturopathic education in Australia. *Complementary Therapies in Australia, 8*, 234–240.

Expert Committee on Complementary Medicines in the Health System. (2003, September). *Complementary medicines in the Australian health system: Report to the parliamentary secretary to the minister of health and ageing.* Canberra, ACT: Australian Government.

Fadlon, J. (2005). *Negotiating the holistic turn: The domestication of alternative medicine.* Albany, NY: State University of New York Press.

Fazari, M. (1999). The role of the chiropractor. *Australasian Chiropractic and Osteopathy, 8*(2), 54–59.

Fechter, S., Wohlmuth, H., Waterman, P., Perdriau, I., Leach, D., & Body, J. (Eds.). (1999, June 16–18). *Herbal medicine into the new millennium conference – Lismore NSW*. Lismore, NSW: Southern Cross University.

Fogliani, C., & Khoury, R. (2003). *Complementary medicine as a model in the Australian healthcare system*. Accessed May 13, 2004, from http://www.acnem.org/journal.

Freidson, E. (1970). *Profession of medicine: A study of the sociology of applied knowledge*. New York: Harper and Row.

Frohock, F. M. (2002). Moving lines and variable criteria: Differences/connections between allopathic and alternative medicine. *The Annals of the American Academy of Political and Social Science, 583*, 214–231.

Fulder, S. (1993). The impact of non-orthodox medicine on our concepts of health. In R. Lafille & S. Fulder (Eds.), *Towards a new science of health* (pp. 105–117). London: Routledge.

Fullagar, S. (2002). Governing the healthy body: Discourses of leisure and lifestyle within Australian health policy. *Health, 6*(1), 69–84.

Gardner, H., & Barraclough, S. (2002). Introduction: Continuity and change in Australian health policy. In H. Gardner & S. Barracligh (Eds.), *Health Policy in Australia* (2nd ed., pp. 1–10). South Melbourne: Oxford University Press.

Gassib-Spain, L., Stewart, A., Tranter, S., & Young, J. (2001). *Complementary therapies and nursing practice: A resource manual for the development of policy*. South East Health, NSW: Southern Eastern Sydney Health Service.

Gawler, I. (2006). Is palliative treatment terminal? A challenging examination of the integrated approach to cancer treatment. In M. Cohen (Ed.), *Holistic health care perspectives* (pp. 120–143). Melbourne, VIC: Australasian Integrative Medicine Association.

Germov, J. (2002). Challenges to medical dominance. In J. Germov (Ed.), *Second opinion: An introduction to health sociology* (pp. 283–305). Melbourne: Oxford University Press.

Gibbon, R. W. (1980). The evolution of chiropractic: Medical and social protest. In S. Haldemann (Ed.), *Modern developments in the principles and practice of chiropractic* (pp. 3–24). New York: Appleton and Lange.

Gillespie, J. A. (1991). *The price of health: Australian governments and medical politics 1910–1960*. Cambridge: Cambridge University Press.

Grace, S., Vemulpad, S., & Beirman, R. (2007). Primary contact practitioner training: A comparison of chiropractic and naturopathic curricula in Australia. *Chiropractic Journal of Australia, 37*(1), 19–24.

Gray, D. E. (2006). *Health sociology: An Australian perspective*. Frenchs Forest, NSW: Pearson Education Australia.

Guthrie, H. N. (1961). *Report of the honorary royal commission appointed to enquire into the provisions of the natural therapists bill – Western Australia*. Perth: Alex B. Davies, Government Printer.

Hadley, C. M. (1988). Complementary medicine and the general practitioner: A survey of general practitioners in the Wellington area. *New Zealand Medical Journal, 101*, 766–768.

Hale, A. (2002). *National survey of naturopaths, herbalists and acupuncturists.* Faculty of Health Sciences, University of Sydney.

Hall, D. (1998). The original structure of ATMS. *Journal of the Australian Traditional Medicine Society, 4*(4), 119–120.

Hall, J., & Viney, R. (2000). The political economy of health sector reform. In A. Bloom (Ed.), *Health reform in Australia and New Zealand* (pp. 39–53). Melbourne: Oxford University Press.

Han, G. S. (2000). Traditional herbal medicine in the Korean community in Australia: A strategy to cope with health demands of immigrant life. *Health, 4*(4), 426–454.

Hancock, L. (1999). Rights and markets: What makes sustainable health policy? In L. Hancock (Ed.), *Health policy in the market state* (pp. 1–15). St. Leonards, NSW: Allen & Unwin.

Hancock, L. (2002). Australian federalism, politics, and health. In H. Gardner & S. Barraclough (Eds.), *Health policy in Australia* (2nd ed., pp. 49–78). Melbourne: Oxford University.

Harries, R. A. (2000). Craniosacral therapy. In R. A. Charman (Ed.), *Complementary therapies for physical therapists* (pp. 144–154). Oxford: Butterworth Heinemann.

Harris, J. (2002). Complementary medicine education: Keeping your distance. *Journal of the Australian Traditional-Medicine Society, 8*(2), 59–61.

Hawkins, P., & O'Neill, A. (1990). *Osteopathy in Australia.* Bundoora, VIC: Phillip Institute of Technology Press.

Heinzman, S. (2004). *Alternative healing: What you should know.* Sydney: ACP Publishing.

Hess, D. J. (2004). Medical modernisation, scientific research fields and the epistemic politics of health social movements. *Sociology of Health and Illness, 26*, 695–709.

Hindle, D., & Perkins, R. (2000). Health care financing in Australia and New Zealand. In A. L. Bloom (Ed.), *Health Reform in Australia and New Zealand* (pp. 80–98). South Melbourne: Oxford University Press.

Hughes, P. (1996). Australia's religious profile. In G. D. Bouma (Ed.), *Many religions, all Australians: Religious settlement, identity and cultural diversity* (pp. 29–50). Adelaide: Open Book Publishers.

Hunter, A. (1991). The changing face of naturopathic medicine in Australia. *Journal of Naturopathic Medicine, 2*(1), 53–56.

Hunter, A. (1997). Why do people see natural therapists? A review of the surveys. *Diversity, 1*(10), 15–18.

Hunter, A. (2002). Natural therapies. *Diversity, 2*(7), 40–47. Accessed October 26, 2004, from http://www.healthy.net/library/journals/naturopathic/vol2no1/aroundw.htm.

Jacka, J. (1989). *Frontiers of natural therapies: A bridge between ancient wisdom and new edges of science*. Melbourne: Lothian Publishing.

Jacka, J. (1998). *Natural therapies: The politics and passion – A personal story of a new profession*. Ringwood, VIC: Ringwood Natural Therapies Pty Ltd.

Jacka, J. (2005). Fifty years of change. *Journal of Australian Natural Therapists Association, 20*(2), 9–11.

Jacka, P. A. (1983). A history of naturopathy in Australia. *Journal of the Australian Natural Therapies Association, 1*(1), 1–9.

James, J. (1999). GST and natural therapies: Acupuncture, naturopathy and herbal medicine win exemption. *Diversity, 1*(18), 4–6.

Johanson, V. (1999). *The new complementary health care council of Australia*. Deakin West, ACT: Complementary Healthcare Council of Australia.

Kapferer, J. (1996). *Being all equal: Identity, difference and Australian cultural practice*. Oxford: Berg.

Kerridge, I., Lowe, M., & McPhee, J. (2005). *Ethics and law for the health professions*. Annandale, NSW: Federation Press.

Kermode, S., Myers, S., & Ramsay, L. (1999). Using natural and complementary therapies on NSW's north coast: Results from a new survey. *Diversity, 1*(16), 13–17.

Khoury, R. (1994). Federation of natural and traditional therapists. *Australian Journal of Medical Herbalism, 6*(1), 15.

Khoury, R. (1999). *Senator Tambling's proposed reforms to complementary medicines,* from http://www.atms.com.au.

Khoury, R. (2001a). AMA president calls for evidence and regulation. *Journal of the Australian Traditional-Medicine Society, 7*(2), 49–52.

Khoury, R. (2001b). Setting up clinic: Allcare naturopathic centre, Sydney. *Journal of the Australian Traditional-Medicine Society, 7*(3), 113–115.

Khoury, R. (2002). The herbalist – Regulating complementary practitioners. *Journal of Complementary Medicine, 1*(1), 43.

Kinney, G. (1975). International College of Chiropractic developments. *Journal of the Australian Chiropractors' Association, 9*(1), 26–27.

Kohn, R. (1991). Radical subjectivity in 'self religions' and the problem of authority. In A. W. Black (Ed.), *Religion in Australia: Sociological perspectives* (pp. 133–150). Sydney: Allen & Unwin.

Kohn, R. (1996). Cults and the new age in Australia. In G. D. Bouma (Ed.), *Many religions, all Australian: Religious settlement, identity and cultural diversity* (pp. 149–162). Adelaide: Open Book Publishers.

Krieken, R. van, Smith, P., Habibis, D., McDonald, K., Haralamobos, M., & Holborn, M. (2000). *Sociology: Themes and Perspectives*. Frenchs Forest, NSW: Longman.

Kron, J. (2003). Osteopathy. *Journal of Complementary Medicine, 2*(5), 22–26.

Lange, R. (1999). *May the people live: A history of Maori health development 1900–1920*. Auckland: Auckland University Press.

Larkin, G. (1983). *Occupational monopoly and modern medicine*. London: Tavistock.

Lawrence, A. (2002). Chiropractic. *Journal of Complementary Medicine, 1*(1), 26–30.

Lawson-Te Aho, K. (1996). *Service evaluation of Te Whare Whakapikiora o te Rangimarie: A Maori traditional healing service* (An Interim Report). Wellington: Te Aho Associates.

Leibrich, J., Hickling, J., & Pitt, G. (1987). *In search of well-being: Exploratory research into complementary therapies*. Wellington: Department of Health.

Levin, J. S., & Coreil, J. (1986). "New age" healing in the U.S. *Social Science and Medicine, 23*, 889–897.

Lewis, J. R. (2005). *Cults* (2nd ed.). Santa Barbara, CA: ABC Clio.

Lewis, M. (1999). World experts to map herbal medicine's future: International conference at Southern Cross University. *Diversity, 1*(17), 21–23.

Lin, V. (2004). The regulation of complementary health: Sacrificing integrity? *Medical Journal of Australia, 180*(2), 96.

Lin, V., Bensoussan, A., Myers, S. P., McCabe, P., Cohen, M., Hill, S., et al. (2005). *The practice and regulatory requirements of naturopathy and Western herbal medicine*. Bundoora, VIC: School of Public Health, La Trobe University.

Lloyd, P. D., Lupton, D., Wiesner, D., & Hasleton, S. (1993). Choosing alternative therapy: An exploratory study of sociodemographic characteristics and motives of patients resident in Sydney. *Australian Journal of Public Health, 17*(2), 135–144.

Lloyd, P. J. (1994). A history of medical professionalisation in NSW, 1788–1950. *Australian Health Review, 17*(2), 14–28.

Locke, R. G. (1993). Who am I in the city of Mammon? The self, doubt and certainty in a Spiritualist cult. In A. W. Black & P. E. Glasner (Eds.), *Sociology of Australian religion* (pp. 108–133). Sydney: Allen & Unwin.

Lucas, N., & Moran, R. (2003). Osteopathy. In T. Robson (Ed.), *An introduction to complementary medicine* (pp. 263–275). Crows Nest, NSW: Allen & Unwin.

Lueng, B. (2008). *Traditional Chinese medicine: The human dimension*. Maleny, QLD: Verdant House.

MacLennan, A. H., Myers, S. P., & Taylor, A. W. (2006). The continuing use of complementary and alternative medicine in South Australia; costs and beliefs in 2004. *Medical Journal of Australia, 184*(1), 27–31.

MacLennan, A. H., Wilson, D. H., & Taylor, A. W. (1996). Prevalence and cost of alternative medicine in Australia. *Lancet, 347*, 569–573.

MacLennan, A. H., Wilson, D. H., & Taylor, A. W. (2002). The escalating cost and prevalence of alternative medicine. *Preventive Medicine, 35*, 166–173.

Maddocks, W. (1995). Safe practice and aromatherapy. *Kai Tiaki: Nursing in New Zealand, 1*(10), 15–16.

Manderson, L., & Matthews, M. (1981). Vietnamese attitudes toward maternal and infant health. *Medical Journal of Australia*, *1*(2), 69–72.

Manderson, L., & Matthews, M. (1985). Care and conflict: Vietnamese medical beliefs and the Australian health care system. In I. Barclay, S. Encel & G. McCall. *Immigration and ethnicity in the 1980s*. Melbourne: Longman-Cheshire.

Manocha, R. (2001). Researching meditation: Clinical applications in health-care. *Diversity*, *2*(5), 3–10.

Marshall, R. J., Gee, R., Israel, M., Neave, D., Edwards, F., Dumble, J., et al. (1990). The use of alternative therapies by Auckland general practitioners. *New Zealand Medical Journal*, *103*(889), 213–215.

Martyr, P. (2002). *Paradise of quacks: An alternative history of medicine in Australia*. Paddington, NSW: Macleay Press.

Martyr, P. (n.d.). From quackery to qualification: Massage and electrotherapy in Australia, 1870–1914. *Electronic Journal of Australian and New Zealand History*. Accessed October 20, 2004, from http://www.jcu.edu.au/aff/history/articles/therapy.htm.

McAllister, W. J. (1976). *The Australian chiropractor*. Beverley SA: Eureka Press.

McCabe, P. (Ed.). (2001). *Complementary therapies in nursing and midwifery: From vision to practice*. Melbourne: Ausmed Publications.

McCabe, P. (2005a). Complementary and alternative medicine in Australia: A contemporary overview. *Complementary Therapies in Clinical Practice*, *11*, 28–31.

McCabe, P. (2005b). Tertiary education in naturopathy and Western herbal medicine. In V. Lin, et al. (Eds.), *The practice and regulatory requirements of naturopathy and Western herbal medicine* (pp. 118–156). Bundoora, VIC: School of Public Health, La Trobe University.

McCutcheon, P. (2003, April 29). *Complementary therapies scrutinised*. Accessed October 20, 2004, from http://www.abc.net.au.

McGregor, K. J., & Peay, E. R. (1996). The choice of alternative therapy for health care: Testing some propositions. *Social Science and Medicine*, *43*, 1317–1327.

McGregor, P. (2000). 'Put yourself in nature's hands': A history of complementary medicine in Victoria. *Diversity*, *2*(2), 12–19.

McGregor, P. (2003). Panic: The media's role in a natural 'product' disaster. *Diversity*, *2*(9), 16–20.

McIver, K. (1997). *Public opinion poll 1997*. Auckland: New Zealand Charter of Health Practitioners.

McQueen, D. (1978). The history of science and medicine as theoretical sources for the comparative study of contemporary medical systems. *Social Science and Medicine*, *12*, 69–74.

Melton, J. G., Clark, J., & Kelly, A. A. (1991). *The new age almanac*. New York: Visible Ink.

Ministerial Advisory Committee on Complementary and Alternative Health. (2004, June). *Complementary and alternative health care in New Zealand: Advice to the minister of health.*

Ministry of Health. (1997). *Taking the pulse: 1996/97 New Zealand health survey.* Wellington: Ministry of Health.

Miskelly, P. A. (2006, July). Healing pluralism and responsibility: An anthropological study of patient and practitioner beliefs. PhD thesis, Waikato University, Hamilton, New Zealand.

Mitchell, D. (2008, January/February). The broad church of medical acupuncture. *Complementary Medicine*, p. 20.

Moore, J. S. (1993). *Chiropractic in America: The history of a medical alternative.* Baltimore, MD: Johns Hopkins University Press.

Morton, M., & Morton, M. (1996). *Five steps to selecting the best alternative medicine: A guide to complementary and integrative health care.* Novato, CA: New World Library.

Moynihan, R. (1999). Widening the options: From a sickness industry to a true health care system. *Diversity, 17*, 4–9.

Murchie, E. (1984). *Rapuora health and Maori women.* Wellington: Maori Women's Welfare League.

Myers, S. P. (2003). Conclusion: Challenges facing integrated medicine. In T. Robson (Ed.), *An introduction to complementary medicine* (pp. 296–308). Crows Nest, NSW: Allen & Unwin.

Myers, S. P. (2006). The legitimacy of traditional medicine: Sorting out anecdotes, empiricism and evidence. In M. Cohen (Ed.), *Holistic healthcare perspectives* (pp. 177–182). Melbourne: Australasian Integrative Medicine Association.

Myers, S. P., Hunter, A., Snider, P., & Zeff, J. L. (2003). Naturopathic medicine. In T. Robson (Ed.), *An introduction to complementary medicine* (pp. 48–66). Crows Nest, NSW: Allen & Unwin.

Najman, J. M. (2003). Health and illness. In I. McAllister, S. Dowrick & R. Hassan (Eds.), *The Cambridge handbook of social sciences in Australia* (pp. 536–553). Cambridge: Cambridge University Press.

National Academic Standards Committee for Traditional Chinese Medicine. (2001). *Australian guidelines for traditional Chinese medicine education.* West End, QLD: Australian Acupuncture and Chinese Medicine Association.

National Association of Naturopaths of Australia. (1975, January). *A submission to the federal committee of inquiry into chiropractic, osteopathy, and naturopathy.*

National Health and Medical Research Council, et al. (2006). *Complementary medicine: Future Directions Forum – Record of proceedings.* Canberra, ACT: Australian Government.

National Institute of Integrative Medicine. (2007). *Study at NIIM, National Institute of Integrative Medicine.* Accessed January 20, 2007, from http://www.niim.com.au.

Natural Health Care Alliance. (2004, February). *NHCA workshop response to the report recommendations of the expert committee on complementary medicines in the health system*. Cremorne, NSW: NHCA.

Navarro, V. (1986). *Crisis, health, and medicine: A social critique*. New York: Tavistock.

Neuenfeldt, K. (1998). The quest for a 'magical island': The convergence of the Didjeridu, Aboriginal culture, healing and cultural politics in New Age discourse. *Social Analysis, 42*(2), 73–97.

New Zealand Consumers' Institute. (1997). From arsenic to zinc. *Consumer, 363,* 20–27.

New Zealand Health Workforce. (2001). *A stocktake of capacity and issues*. Wellington: New Zealand Ministry of Health.

Ngu, M. (1998). The Australian Integrative Medicine Association. *Diversity, 1*(15) 25–26.

NSWHEALTH. (2002). *Regulation of complementary health practitioners – Discussion paper*, from http://www.health.nsw.gov.au.

O'Brien, K. (2004). Complementary and alternative medicine: The move into mainstream health care. *Clinical and Experimental Optometry, 87*(2), 110–120.

O'Callaghan, F. V., & Jordan, N. (2003). Postmodern values, attitudes, and use of complementary medicine. *Complementary Therapies in Medicine, 11*(1), 353–58.

O'Neill, A. (1994a). *Enemies within and without: Educating chiropractors, osteopaths, and traditional acupuncturists*. Bundoora, VIC: La Trobe University Press.

O'Neill, A. (1994b). Danger and safety in medicine. *Social Science and Medicine, 38,* 497–507.

O'Neill, A. (1995). Daylight at noon: Alternative health battles. In H. Gardner (Ed.), *The politics of health: The Australian experience* (pp. 428–451). Melbourne: Churchill Livingstone.

O'Reilly, B. K. (1981). Chiropractic education in Australia. *Chiropractic Australia, 1*(1), 10–12.

Osteopathy House. (n.d.). *New South Wales College of Osteopathy*. Sydney: Osteopathy House.

Owen, D., & Lewith, G. T. (2004). Teaching integrated care: CAM familiarisation courses. *Medical Journal of Australia, 181*(5), 276–278.

Parker, M. H. (2003). The regulation of complementary health: Sacrificing integrity. *Medical Journal of Australia, 179*(6), 316–318.

Pearson, B. (2002). Gathering the profession together. *Journal of the Traditional-Medicine Society, 8*(4), 157–159.

Pearson, B., & Khoury, R. (2003). Complementary medicine practitioner associations council (CMPAC). *Journal of the Australian Traditional-Medicine Society, 9*(1), 39–40.

Pensabene, T. S. (1980). *The rise of the medical practitioner in Victoria* [Health Research Project, Research Monograph 2]. Canberra, ACT: Australian National University.

Peter, J. J., & Associates (2000, July). *Vocational education and training opportunities within the WA complementary therapies industry: Final report.* Report prepared for the Western Australian Department of Training and Employment – Strategic Services Division.

Peters, D., & Woodham, A. (2000). *The complete guide to integrated medicine: The best of complementary and conventional care*, St. Leonards, NSW: Dorling Kindersley.

Peters, R. E., & Peters, M. A. (1986). Chiropractic in Australia in 1985: A thumbnail sketch. *European Journal of Chiropractic, 33*, 169–187.

Petersen, A. (1994a). *In a critical condition: Health and power relations in Australia.* St. Leonards, NSW: Allen & Unwin.

Petersen, A. (1994b). Risk, governance and the new public health. In A. Petersen & R. Bunton (Eds.), *Foucault, health and medicine* (pp. 189–226). London: Routledge.

Phelps, K. (2003). *Doctors, healing, and the role of complementary medicine.* Australian Medical Association, accessed September 15, 2004, from http://www.ama.com.au/web.nsf/doc/WEEN-5MT8UY.

Phillips, P. J. (1978). *Kill or cure: Lotions, potions, characters and quacks of early Australia.* Richmond, VIC: Greenhouse Publications.

Pietroni, P. C. (1992). Beyond the boundaries: Relationship between general practice and complementary medicine. *British Medical Journal, 305,* 564–565.

Pirotta, M. V., Cohen, M. C., Kotsirilos, V., & Farish, S. J. (2000). Complementary therapies: Have they become accepted in general practice? *Medical Journal of Australia, 172,* 105–109.

Pizzorno, J. E., Jr. (1996). Naturopathic medicine. In M. S. Micozzi (Ed.), *Fundamentals of complementary and alternative medicine* (pp. 163–181). New York: Churchill Livingston.

Podger, A., & Hagan, P. (2000). Reforming the Australian health care system: The role of government. In A. Bloom (Ed.) *Health reform in Australia and New Zealand* (pp. 115–131). Melbourne: Oxford University Press.

Portelli, M. (1985). Looking back at chiropractic in Australia. *Chiropractic Australia, 5*(2), 13–17.

Possamai, A. (2000). A profile of new agers: Social and spiritual aspects. *Journal of Sociology, 36*(3), 364–377.

Powell, C. (2003). *Anatomy of the Australian natural medicine industry: Future opportunities.* Brisbane: Report prepared for the Australian College of Natural Medicine.

Poynton, L., Dowell, A., Dew, K., & Egan, T. (2006). General practitioners' attitudes toward (and use of) complementary and alternative medicine: A New Zealand nationwide survey. *New Zealand Medical Journal, 119*(1247), 1–10.

Prince, R., & Riches, D. (2000). *The new age in Glastonbury: The construction of religious movements.* New York: Berghahn.

Pruss, W. (2006). Natural therapies from the 1890s to 1950s. *The Natural Therapist*, 21(1), 31–33.

Quinn, F. (2006). *Community and alternative medicine in New Zealand*. Winston Churchill Memorial Trust Travelling Fellowship Report. Wellington: Winston Church Memorial Fellowship Trust.

Ravenhill, J. (1993). Business and politics. In R. Smith (Ed.), *Politics in Australia* (2nd ed., pp. 262–284). St. Leonards, NSW: Allen & Unwin.

Rayner, L., & Easthope, G. (2001). Postmodern consumption and alternative medications. *Journal of Sociology*, 37(2), 157–176.

Reader, W. L., & Bryner, P. (1989). The development of chiropractic in New Zealand, 1910–1980. *Chiropractic History*, 9, 17–21.

Reid, J. (1983). *Sorcerers and healing spirits: Continuity and change in an Aboriginal community*. Canberra, ACT: Australian National University Press.

Richards, D. (1994). To minister to the sick: An historic socio-profile of the medical profession in Northern Australia. In J. Pearn (Ed.), *Outback medicine: Some vignettes of pioneering medicine* (pp. 23–42). Brisbane: Amphon Press.

Robson, T. (Ed.) (2003). *An introduction to complementary medicine*. Crows Nest, NSW: Allen & Unwin.

Roth, J. A. (1976). *Health purifiers and their enemies: A study of the natural health movement in the United States with a comparison to its counterpart in Germany*. New York: Prodist.

Rubin, H. (1999). Creating the herb growing industry. In S. Fechter, et al. (Eds.), *Herbal medicine into the new millennium – Lismore NSW 16–18 June 1999* (pp. 11–14). Lismore, NSW: Southern Cross University.

Saks, M. (2003). *Orthodox and alternative medicine: Politics, professionalization, and health care*. New York: Continuum.

Scott, A. L. (1999). Paradoxes of holism: Some problems in developing an anti-oppressive medical practice. *Health*, 3(2), 131–149.

Sedmond, S. (1999). Global herbalism cross-pollinates: A herbalist's impression of the herbal medicine into the new millennium conference. *Diversity*, 1(18), 12–13.

Sherwood, P. (2000). Patterns of use of complementary health services in the south-west of Western Australia. *Australian Journal of Rural Health*, 8, 194–200.

Sherwood, P. (2004). Evolution of natural medicine and biomedicine and their future roles in health care. PhD thesis, Faculty of Human Development, Victoria University, Melbourne, Australia.

Sherwood, P. (2005). *Healing: The history, philosophy and practice of natural medicine*. Brisbane: Australian College of Natural Medicine.

Siahpush, M. (1998). Postmodern values, dissatisfaction with conventional medicine and popularity of alternative therapies. *Journal of Sociology*, 34, 58–70.

Siahpush, M. (1999). A critical review of the sociology of alternative medicine: Research on users, practitioners, and the orthodoxy. *Health*, *4*(2), 159–178.

News and Comment. (2003). One nation's victory for sanity over alternative medicine. *Skeptical Inquirer*, *27*(5), 1–2.

Social Development Committee. (1986). *Inquiry into alternative medicine and the health food industry* (Vol. 1). Melbourne: Parliament of Victoria.

Spitzer, O. (2002). The role of the therapeutic relationship. *Diversity*, *2*(7), 17–23.

Sprarrow, J., & Sprarrow, J. (2001). *Radical Melbourne: A secret history*. Carlton North, VIC: Vulgar Press.

Stannard, G. (2002, August 2). *The art and the science of naturopathy: An Australian perspective*. *Science – New Wave*. Accessed July 15, 2005, from http://nextwave.sciencemag.org.

Stone, J., & Heller, T. (2005). Cash and CAM: The private sector and CAM practice. In T. Heller, G. Lee-Treweek, J. Katz, J. Stone & S. Spurr (Eds.), *Perspectives in complementary and alternative medicine* (pp. 353–378). Abdingdon, OX: Routledge.

Sutton, J. (2004). Homebirth as an alternative to the dominative system of hospital birth in Australia, from http://www.maternitycoalition.org.au.

Sweaney, J. A. (1989). History of the Australian Chiropractors' Association: The first twenty-five years. *Chiropractic History*, *9*, 31–36.

Szymanski, A. J., & Goertzel, T. G. (1979). *Sociology: Class, consciousness, and contradictions*. New York: D. Van Nostrand.

Taylor, J. M. (1973). *Southern school of naturopathy – Report for naturopathic, osteopathic and chiropractic inquiry*. Melbourne: Southern School of Naturopathy.

Templeton, J. (1969). *Prince Henry's: The evolution of a Melbourne Hospital*. Melbourne: Robertson and Mullins.

Te Pumanawa Hauora. (1997). *Oranga Kaumatua: The health and wellbeing of older Maori people*. A Report Prepared for the Ministries of Health and Maori Development, Maori Studies, Massey University, Palmerston North, New Zealand.

Teschendorff, J. (2001). Does holistic medicine ignore the social causes of illness? *Diversity*, *2*(4), 46–51.

Tippens, K., & Connelly, E. (2007). 'Poverty and human development': The social responsibility of the naturopathic physician. *Journal of Alternative and Complementary Medicine*, *13*, 783–785.

Tiqua, R. C. (2004). *Traditional Chinese medicine as an Australian tradition of health care*. PhD thesis, History and Philosophy of Science, University of Melbourne, Australia.

Trevenna, J., & Reeder, A. (2005, December 16). Perceptions of New Zealand adults about complementary and alternative therapies for cancer treatment. *New Zealand Medical Journal*, *118*(1227), 1–11.

Trowbridge, C. (1991). *Andrew Taylor still, 1828–1917*. Kirksville, MO: Thomas Jefferson University Press.

Tuchtan, V. M. (2003). Massage therapy. In T. Robson (Ed.), *An introduction to complementary therapy* (pp. 229–244). Crows Nest, NSW: Allen & Unwin.

University of Queensland News Online. (2003, November 19). *Call for health professionals to be more educated on complementary medicine* (p. 1), from http://www.uq.edu.au/news.

Waitzkin, H. (2000). *The second sickness: Contradictions of capitalist health care*. Lanham, MD: Rowman & Littlefield.

Ward, H. R. (1975). *Report from the osteopathy, chiropractic and naturopathy committee*. Melbourne: C.H. Rixon, Government Printer.

Wearing, M. (2004). Medical dominance and the division of labour in the health professions. In C. Grbich (Ed.), *Health in Australia: Sociological concepts and issues* (3rd ed., pp. 260–289). Frenchs Forest, NSW: Pearson Longman.

Weir, M. (2000a). Who can practice complementary medicine? The need for legal reform. *Diversity*, *2*(3), 26–32.

Weir, M. (2000b). *Complementary medicine: Ethics and law*. Brisbane: Prometheus.

Weir, M. (2005). *Alternative medicine: A new regulatory model*. Melbourne: Australian Scholarly.

White, K. N. (1999). Negotiating science and liberalism: Medicine in nineteenth-century South Australia. *Medical History*, *43*, 173–191.

White, K. N. (2000–2001). What's happening in general practice: Capitalist monopolisation and state administrative control: A profession bailing out? *Annual Review of Health Social Sciences*, *10*, 5–18.

White, K. N. (2002). *An introduction to the sociology of health and illness*. London: Sage.

Whyte, S. R., van der Geest, S., & Hardon, A. (2002). *Social lives of medicines*. Cambridge: Cambridge University Press.

Wiesner, D. (1981). Sociological aspects of naturopathy. Thesis, University of Adelaide, South Australia.

Wiesner, D. (1989). *Alternative medicine: A guide for patients and health professionals in Australia*. Kenthurst, NSW: Kangaroo Press.

Wilkinson, J. M., & Simpson, M. D. (2001). High use of complementary health services in a New South Wales country town. *Australian Journal of Rural Health*, *9*, 166–171.

Williams, B. (2003). One nation's victory for sanity over alternative medicine. *Skeptical Inquirer*, *27*, 5. Accessed November 5, 2004, from http://www.skeptics.com.au.

Williams, N. (2004, February 14). Naturopaths warned over bad medicine. *The Daily Telegraph*, p. 17.

Willis, E. (1988). Doctoring in Australia: A view at the bicentenary. *Milbank Quarterly*, *66*, 167–181.

Willis, E. (1989a). *Medical dominance: The division of labour in Australian health care*. St. Leonards, NSW: Allen & Unwin.

Willis, E. (1989b). Complementary healers. In G. M. Lupton & J. M. Najman (Eds.), *Sociology of health and illness: Australian readings* (pp. 259–267). South Melbourne: MacMillan.

Willis, E. (1991). Chiropractic in Australia. *Journal of Manipulative and Physiological Therapeutics, 14*(1), 60.

Willis, E. (1993). Chiropractic and osteopathy at the crossroads: Opening address to COMSIG Chiropractic Conference. *COMSIG Review, 2*(1), 1–4.

Willis, E., & White, K. (2004). Evidence-based medicine and CAM. In P. Tovey, G. Easthope & J. Adams (Eds.), *Mainstreaming complementary and alternative medicine: Studies in social context* (pp. 49–63). London: Routledge.

Winter, D. O. (1975, January). *A submission on chiropractic by the Australian chiropractors' association to the Federal Committee of Enquiry into Chiropractic, Osteopathy and Naturopathy*. Australian Chiropractors' Association.

Wiseman, J. (1998). *Global nation? Australia and the politics of globalisation*. Cambridge: Cambridge University Press.

Wohlmuth, H. (2003). Herbal medicine. In T. Robson (Ed.), *An introduction to complementary medicine* (pp. 191–212). Crows Nest, NSW: Allen & Unwin.

Woodham, A., & Peters, D. (1997). *Encyclopedia of natural healing: The definitive reference guide to treatments for mind and body*. St. Leonards, NSW: Dorling Kindersley.

Woodham, A., & Peters, D. (1997). *The encyclopedia of natural healing: The definitive Australian reference guide*. St. Leonards, NSW: Dorling Kindersley.

Woodward, D. (2002). Economic policy. In J. Summers, D. Woodward & A. Parkin (Eds.), *Government, politics, power and policy in Australia* (7th ed., pp. 417–438). Frenchs Forest, NSW. Longman.

World Health Organization. (2001). *Legal status of traditional medicine and complementary medicine: A worldwide review*. Geneva: WHO.

Xue, C. C. L., Zhang, A. L., Lin, V., Da Costa, C., & Story, D. F. (2007). Complementary and alternative medicine use in Australia: A national population-survey. *Journal of Alternative and Complementary Medicine, 6*, 643–650.

York, M. (1995). *The emerging network: A sociology of new age and neo-pagan movements*. Lanham, MD: Rowman & Littlefield.

SUBJECT INDEX

Printed and bound by CPI Group (UK) Ltd, Croydon, CR0 4YY

17/10/2024

01775697-0002